640104 D0269059

Fertility

Fertility

Dr Elizabeth Clubb
and
Jane Knight

Charts and diagrams by
Oxford Medical Illustrations,
John Radcliffe Hospital

David & Charles

ABOUT THE AUTHORS

Dr Elizabeth Clubb and **Jane Knight** are a doctor and nurse team with many years' experience teaching natural family planning methods to women, couples and health professionals. As Medical Director and National Tutor respectively of the Natural Family Planning Service, they are also extensively involved in researching, writing and lecturing in this field.

A DAVID & CHARLES BOOK

First published in the UK in 1987
Reprinted 1988
Second edition published 1992
This edition published 1996

Copyright © Dr Elizabeth Clubb and Jane Knight 1987, 1992, 1996

Dr Elizabeth Clubb and Jane Knight have asserted their right to be identified as authors of this work in accordance with the Copyright, Designs and Patents Act, 1988.

All rights reserved. No part of this publication may be reproduced, stored in a retrieval system, or transmitted, in any form or by any means, electronic or mechanical, by photocopying, recording or otherwise, without prior permission in writing from the publisher.

A catalogue record for this book is available from the British Library.

ISBN 0 7153 0424 0

Book design and typesetting by Les Dominey Design Company, Exeter
and printed in England by Redwood Books
for David & Charles
Brunel House   Newton Abbot   Devon

Contents

Acknowledgements 6

Foreword 7

Introduction 9

1. Fertility awareness 12

The sympto-thermal method 15

2. Reproductive anatomy and physiology 15

3. The first indicator – temperature 33

4. The second indicator – cervical mucus 41

5. Factors affecting the menstrual cycle 52

6. The third indicator – cervix 58

7. Minor indicators of fertility 62

8. Use of a calendar calculation 66

9. Planning a family by the sympto-thermal method 70

10. Effectiveness 77

Fertility awareness and NFP in special circumstances 82

11. After childbirth and during breast-feeding 82

12. Post-pill users 95

13. The pre-menopausal years 103

Gynaecology 118

14. Infertility and subfertility 118

15. Contraception, sterilisation and abortion 128

16. Vaginal infections, sexually transmitted diseases and cancer 145

17. Scientific research and new technologies 152

Teaching 159

18. Teaching fertility awareness and natural family planning 159

     Living with natural family planning 166

Appendix 168

     Information which can be gained from the sympto-thermal chart 168

     Sympto-thermal chart 170

     Instructions for use of the sympto-thermal chart 171

Addresses 172

Bibliography 173

Glossary 176

Index 190

ACKNOWLEDGEMENTS

The authors would like to thank the following:

John Marshall who pioneered the temperature method and established the first organisation to teach natural family planning in the UK.

John Bonnar for his encouragement and time spent in reading and correcting the manuscript.

Victoria Jennings and Virginia Lamprecht, from The Institute of Reproductive Health, Georgetown University, USA for their support of innovative projects and international research and particularly to Cecilia Pyper, Consultant to the Institute, for her assistance in updating this edition.

Sian Martin and our colleagues in the NFP Service for posing the questions that we have tried to answer in this book.

Anna Flynn, Colleen Norman, and our colleagues in the National Association of NFP Teachers for their expertise and co-operation.

Suzanne Parenteau Carreau and other members of SERENA, Canada who have shared their experiences in teaching breast-feeding women.

John and Evelyn Billings for their work in the development of the Ovulation method.

Sarah Rowland-Jones, for her HIV research and Peter Jones for his advice in updating the section on HIV and AIDS.

And John and Peter for their tireless technological support.

FOREWORD

This book will be of great interest and help to women and to couples who wish to know about fertility and to understand the principles of natural family planning. A great deal of misinformation persists among health care workers about natural family planning, and this book should be essential reading for doctors, nurses and others who advise on the subject.

In the last twenty-five years, largely due to the efforts of the World Health Organisation, major advances have occurred in our understanding of fertility and the process of ovulation. Among couples practising birth control, between 5 and 25 per cent use some form of natural family planning. Worldwide usage is estimated at thirty-one million couples.

In the context of family planning, the term 'natural' is used to describe methods of fertility control which are based on the recognition and interpretation of physiological or natural markers which determine the fertile and infertile phases in each menstrual cycle. Concern about both the side-effects and the high discontinuation rates with hormonal contraception have reinforced the need for providing couples with accurate information on natural family planning. Many couples, given the opportunity, express a preference for a natural method of family planning but to be successful, both partners need to be well motivated. A clear understanding of the whole subject of fertility, and the methods of natural family planning, such as will be gained from reading this book, will provide couples with the confidence they need.

Current methods of natural family planning are based on the concept of fertility awareness and the woman's ability to identify on a day-to-day basis certain changes in her body related to its preparation for ovulation. Early studies carried out by the World Health Organisation show that virtually all women can learn to detect the fertile and infertile times of their cycle irrespective of their level of education. Natural family planning involves a learning process and aims to make the users both independent, and potential educators of other users. In contrast to oral contraceptives and intra-uterine devices, it does not require medical intervention and supervision.

Dr Elizabeth Clubb and Jane Knight have extensive experience in education for natural family planning. Their book provides an excellent review of the current methods of natural family planning and their use in special circumstances such as following childbirth, during breast-feeding, after coming off the pill and when approaching the menopause. The authors provide a highly readable account of the factual information on human reproduction which forms the scientific basis for the cycle of fertility. They discuss the latest research into natural family planning and its implications for the use of these methods.

Natural family planning can be used both to achieve and to avoid pregnancy. The book includes a review of infertility and the use of fertility awareness to assist in improving the chances of pregnancy, and discusses the investigations recommended for the couple with infertility. A comprehensive account is also given of the existing methods of contraception, sterilisation, abortion and sexually transmitted disease.

I recommend this book to all who are engaged in the health care and education of women and those providing family planning services.

John Bonnar.

John Bonnar, MA, MD, FRCOG
Professor of Obstetrics and Gynaecology
Trinity College University of Dublin

INTRODUCTION

Our fertility is one of our greatest gifts. In many parts of the less developed world, a man's children are still his wealth. He looks to them to work for him in sickness and old age. They are his Welfare State. Family planning for him means having many children. But there is another side to this coin. As populations grow, and outstrip resources, so do the social and economic pressures. In the past when striving to live in harmony with the environment, measures had to be taken to limit the size of families and of the tribe. In parts of the world where harsh climates prevailed and food supplies were scarce, desperate measures were resorted to, and infants were exposed to the elements and the old and ailing were left to die. Other populations were controlled by laws governing the relationship between men and women, and taboos which controlled the timing and frequency of sexual intercourse.

In the developing world as well as in Europe and the USA, young couples today face social and economic problems when they assume parental responsibilities. So family planning is about having children, as well as about avoiding pregnancy. It is about deciding when to start a family, the number of children and how they should be spaced, according to circumstances. In a recent survey, women were asked to describe the 'ideal' family planning method. High on the list were: No side effects (62 per cent), followed by Reliable (59 per cent) and Natural (39 per cent).

Natural methods of family planning have been researched and developed for the purpose of finding an efficient and reliable method acceptable to peoples of different cultures and religions. The search has been to develop a method that was without health hazards and one that would help couples to conceive as well as to avoid pregnancy and therefore to be in control of their own fertility. The importance of the research work carried out during the last 60 years lies in the fact that a scientific basis for these methods has been discovered; and that from this knowledge, accurate guidelines for identifying the fertile and infertile phases of a woman's cycle are now available.

It is interesting to learn from World Health Organisation personnel engaged in teaching natural family planning that many peoples in Arabia, Africa, and South East Asia are aware of the rhythms of fertility and infertility occurring during the menstrual cycle. This tradition has been passed down from mother to daughter. Much of this research work has therefore resulted in rediscovery for Western civilisation of folklore well known in the East.

THE HISTORY OF NATURAL FAMILY PLANNING

SINGLE-INDEX METHODS

The Rhythm or Calendar Method

The first natural method was discovered in 1929 by Dr Knaus in Austria, who observed that ovulation occurred at a fixed time of around 14 days before the next menstrual period. In 1930 Dr Ogino in Japan made a similar observation independently. This knowledge formed the basis of the rhythm method in which calculations were made to predict the fertile and infertile phases of the cycle. This method is still being practised in some countries, but due to its reliance on regular cycles and the long period of abstinence required, it is less effective than more modern methods and is not widely used.

The Temperature Method

In the late 1920s it was observed that a small rise in a woman's basal (waking) body temperature occurred following ovulation due to the influence of the hormone progesterone. In the UK the practical details of the temperature method were worked out by Professor John Marshall.

The Mucus Method

Just as women are aware of blood flow every month during the period, so they can be helped to recognise the flow of mucus which occurs mid-cycle. Although cervical mucus had been observed by women over the centuries, it was not until the late nineteenth century that Sims reported the potential of cervical mucus to block or aid sperm migration. In 1933 changes in cervical mucus were related to a rise in oestrogen levels in the urine prior to ovulation. Using mucus as an indicator of fertility and timing intercourse in relation to mucus changes was mainly the work of Drs John and Evelyn Billings in Australia. This is known as the Billings or Ovulation method of natural family planning and is widely used.

MULTIPLE-INDEX METHODS

The Sympto-thermal Method

The sympto-thermal method combines observations of cervical mucus with temperature readings and other indicators of fertility. This method was variously described as the muco-thermic method (Marshall, UK) and the double-check method (Thyma, USA). It offers a high degree of effectiveness and for this reason detailed information on the sympto-thermal method and a step-by-step guide to achieve or avoid pregnancy forms the major part of this book.

These methods of Natural Family Planning are now taught in more than a hundred countries world-wide, and research goes on into the immensely complicated interaction of women's hormones. This is leading to new technologies for women wishing to use a natural method of family planning.

1. Fertility Awareness

Fertility and reproductive health are largely neglected areas in health education, and this ignorance, and the lack of accurate available information about the increasingly popular methods of natural family planning, means that women are denied the full range of family planning choices open to them.

This ignorance was revealed when the results of a survey carried out in 1993 in six countries in Western Europe found that the majority of women lacked knowledge concerning basic facts about menstruation, fertility and pregnancy (*The Wise Report*, Unipath).

■ One fifth of women had no idea what was happening when their periods started.

■ Europe-wide there was misunderstanding regarding the process of ovulation and the timing of conception.

■ In the UK one third of the women questioned believed that ovulation occurs during menstruation.

■ The number of fertile days in the menstrual cycle was over estimated. In the UK, 21 per cent of women thought that there were more than 21 fertile days (the average number is seven).

Women really need to know the facts about themselves to make sense of the problems which they continue to meet. Fertility awareness is the essential basic education for understanding their fertility from adolescence to the menopause. It can help them to understand human sexuality and reproductive health. It can help them to value their fertility which can be easily damaged by infections, especially sexually transmitted diseases, many of which may lead on to fertility problems. It will also help them to make informed choices on methods of contraception, or can teach them to use a natural method of family planning.

It is very important to recognise that family planning is not just a way to avoid conception and pregnancy. It should aim to enable people to choose whether and when to have a baby, helping them with information about spacing births and infertility advice, especially if they have problems of subfertility. The ideal method of family planning should not harm their health or fertility, and should enhance the enjoyment of their relationship.

Most women rely on medical advice when looking for a method of family planning. It is usually the woman who makes the decision, although from the results contained in the Wise Report, in answer to their questionnaire the majority of women said that they would prefer to share this decision-making with their partner.

FERTILITY AWARENESS IS FUNDAMENTAL TO AN UNDERSTANDING OF FAMILY PLANNING

- For a woman, fertility awareness includes the ability to identify the signs and symptoms of fertility during the menstrual cycle, so that she will know which days she is fertile and which days she is infertile.
- For a man, fertility awareness includes understanding his own reproductive potential.
- For the couple, fertility awareness includes the understanding of their combined fertility at different stages of their lives, and this will give them the knowledge and confidence to make the important decisions concerned with planning a family.

A couple who understand the rhythm of fertility occurring each month will be able to use natural family planning (NFP). An increasing number of women choose a natural method for health or for ecological reasons. It is important for them to know that NFP can be used throughout a woman's fertile life, that it does not rely on regular cycles, and that it can be used after childbirth and during breast-feeding. It can also be used during the pre-menopausal years.

Modern methods of NFP do not rely on 'Rhythm' or 'Calendar Calculations', but are based on a scientific and accurate understanding of fertility – 'Fertility Awareness'. Many women learn NFP in order to achieve pregnancy. As many as one couple in six experience some difficulty in conceiving. Fertility Awareness will help them to maximise their chances of conception before turning to more detailed medical intervention.

Beyond helping them make responsible choices about family planning, a sound awareness of fertility issues can enable a couple, should they choose a natural method, to have absolute and complete control over their own family planning.

FERTILITY AWARENESS CAN HELP COUPLES TOWARDS A BETTER UNDERSTANDING OF EACH OTHER

Although it doesn't guarantee to cure the problem, an understanding of *why* we feel the way we do *when* we do often helps us understand each other better. Many women are mystified by their own physiology. Some days they feel fit and well and capable of tremendous activity, on other days tiredness and a feeling of inability to cope leads to depression. Their bewildered partners may be less than patient with them at these times. Some women experience these mood swings every month, 'pre-menstrual tension', others after having a baby, 'post-natal depression', and others are troubled later in life at the time of the pre-menopause.

The anxiety caused by these physical feelings and emotional swings is magnified by ignorance. If a woman and her partner can learn more about the hormones which play such an important role in her life, and be confident that her experience is natural and will pass, she may be able to cope with them. If the symptoms are severe, she should seek medical advice –

there is much that can be done to help her. Her partner can also benefit from fertility awareness education, which could enable him to understand the cause of her problems. His loving consideration can help them both.

Men and women have a right to learn about the importance of reproductive health and to value their fertility and be able to plan their families. Fertility awareness will help them.

2. Reproductive Anatomy and Physiology

Some knowledge of male and female anatomy is important for each person wishing to learn fertility awareness and so understand natural methods of family planning. When the basic facts are clearly understood, it is easier to see how the fertile and infertile phases of the woman's cycle can be determined and why necessary guidelines are given.

MALE REPRODUCTIVE ORGANS

The male reproductive system is composed of two testicles (testes) from each of which runs a tube, known as the vas deferens, which opens into the urethra. The urethra is the tube which runs through the penis and conveys urine from the bladder to the outside. The seminal vesicles and ducts from the prostate gland also open into the urethra.

The testicles are contained in a special pouch of skin known as the scrotum. At puberty, they begin to function in two ways:

- They produce the male hormone testosterone, which is responsible for the development of male secondary sex characteristics, such as deepening of the voice, growth of the beard and pubic hair.
- They produce male sex cells (spermatozoa, sperm). Together with the female sex cell, or ovum, they are capable of producing new life.

THE TEMPERATURE-REGULATING FUNCTION OF THE SCROTUM
The testes must be at a temperature slightly lower than the rest of the body to produce sperm cells efficiently. If the temperature is too high or too low, sperm cell production is adversely affected.

The scrotum hangs outside the body, between the legs, and serves to control the temperature of the testes. If the temperature is too high, the scrotum gives off heat in two ways: by sweating; and by relaxing its muscle layer so that the surface area expands. In cold temperatures the muscle layer contracts, making the surface area of the scrotum smaller and drawing the testes in closer to the warmth of the body.

Interference with the normal temperature-regulating mechanism may be a contributing factor to male fertility problems. Men working in particularly high temperatures, and men wearing excessively tight clothing, may show a low sperm count.

THE PRODUCTION OF SPERM AND SEMINAL FLUID
Each testis contains a long system of coiled, tightly packed tubules the linings of which produce sperm in a continuous process. The sperm then pass

15

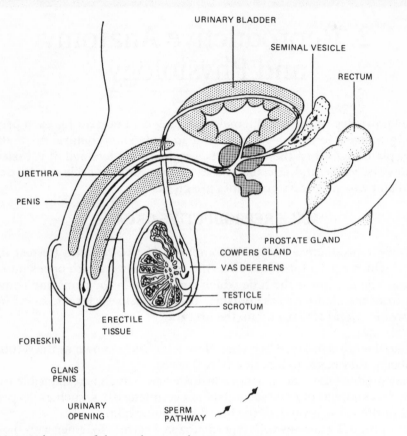

Fig 2.1 Side view of the male reproductive organs

along to the epididymis at the upper part of the testis, where they are stored for about 12 days during which time they gain their motility and their fertilising capacity, thus reaching maturity.

At ejaculation, sperm are propelled through the vas deferens into the urethra where they join secretions from the seminal vesicles and prostate gland. These secretions assist in the preservation and nourishment of the sperm cells, and add volume to make up the seminal fluid or semen. The rhythmic muscular contractions of the tubes leading from the testes to the outside, and the muscular portion of the prostate gland, help to expel the fluid with some force: ejaculation or male orgasm. Between two and five millilitres of seminal fluid containing around 100,000,000 sperm cells per millilitre may be thus released. Only about 100 sperm survive the long and hazardous journey to reach the ovum (female sex cell) and only one sperm will finally penetrate the ovum to achieve fertilisation and pregnancy.

The male urethra forms a common pathway for seminal fluid and urine. There is, however, a complex valve system that ensures the functions of urination and sexual activity leading to ejaculation cannot take place simultaneously.

THE SPERMATOZOON

The spermatozoon or male sex cell is microscopic in size. It comprises a head, middle section or neck, and a tail. The head contains a nucleus with 23 rod-shaped chromosomes. These chromosomes carry the father's genes – his genetic contribution to his child. The middle section contains the energy supply to nourish the sperm and assist in movement. The slender whip-like tail enables the sperm cell to move forward by lashing energetically from side to side.

Mature sperm reach their full motile capacity when they are mixed with fluids from the other sex glands to form the seminal fluid or semen. This is a thick, viscous, whitish and slightly alkaline fluid with a distinct odour. It acts as the medium for transporting sperm to the female genital tract. It must be remembered that a man is always fertile. From the age of puberty (at which time sperm become mature), he may continue to produce viable sperm into the ninth decade of life.

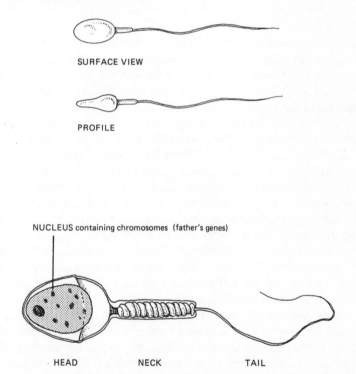

SURFACE VIEW

PROFILE

NUCLEUS containing chromosomes (father's genes)

HEAD   NECK   TAIL

Fig 2.2 Spermatozoa. The head of the sperm is ovoid-shaped but flattened, so that when seen in profile it appears pear-shaped.

PRE-EJACULATORY FLUID

The Cowpers glands secrete a lubricating fluid to prepare the urethra for sperm transport. A few drops of this fluid, which may contain sperm, leak out during sexual excitement and before ejaculation. It must be emphasised that genital contact even without full intercourse, could result in pregnancy in the presence of fertile mucus. The sperm may be attracted into the vagina by the mucus. For this reason coitus interruptus (withdrawal) is not a reliable means of preventing pregnancy. Even if the man withdraws in good time before he ejaculates, the pre-ejaculatory fluid could cause a pregnancy, if there is fertile mucus present at the vaginal entrance.

SPERM SURVIVAL

Sperm may survive in the female reproductive tract for up to 72 hours in the presence of fertile mucus. Longer survival times have been recorded of five or more days, but these are exceptional cases. Sperm may live in the specialised crypts of the woman's cervix, nourished and protected by cervical mucus, thus retaining their capacity to fertilise the ovum.

At times of infertility, when the cervical mucus is thick, forming the mucus plug, which is an impenetrable barrier to sperm, the sperm in the vagina are destroyed within hours by the acidity of the vaginal secretions.

THE PENIS

The shaft of the penis is composed of soft, spongy tissue which is capable of becoming firm during sexual stimulation. When a man is sexually aroused, the arteries in the penis open up to allow increased blood-flow to the penis so that it fills with blood, and becomes firm and erect in preparation for sexual intercourse.

The skin around the penis has a great number of sensitive nerve endings. These are concentrated on the underside of the shaft of the penis, and over the whole surface of the glans. When these nerve endings are stimulated, there is a build-up of sexual tension and erection of the penis. During sexual intercourse, the erect penis is inserted into the vagina – penetration. Sexual tension is normally released at the time of ejaculation when orgasm normally takes place. Following this, the penis returns to its flaccid state.

The glans penis is covered by a separate hood of skin known as the foreskin or prepuce. The foreskin retracts during erection exposing the glans. It is the foreskin which is removed at circumcision. This operation is most commonly performed for cultural or religious reasons, although there are medical reasons for circumcision.

The whole mechanism of erection and ejaculation is a reflex activity. It works most successfully in a state of relaxation. The reflex control can be affected by emotional or mental influences, drugs or alcohol. Physical or emotional stress may therefore result in a man's inability to gain or sustain an erection, and his sexual performance may be affected as a result.

FEMALE EXTERNAL GENITALS (VULVA)

Although the major reproductive organs in the female are internal, in contrast to the external male organs, the female's external genitals or vulva are the counterparts of many of the male organs.

The mons pubis (pubic mound) is a soft, fatty pad lying over and protecting the pubic bone. It is covered by the typically triangular shaped female pubic hair. The mons continues backwards to form the labia majora (outer lips) of the vulva. These are soft folds extending backwards to just in front of the anal area. They develop from the same embryological tissue as the male scrotum.

Inside the outer lips are the labia minora (inner lips) of the vulva. These are thinner, smooth and silky. They are the female counterpart of tissue that forms the shaft of the male penis. The inner lips contain numerous sensitive nerve endings. During sexual stimulation the labia become engorged with blood like the shaft of the penis and the inner lips become moist.

The labia minora unite at the front around the clitoris. The clitoris is a small knob of highly sensitive erectile tissue (the female counterpart of the male glans penis). It is covered by a prepuce or hood which corresponds to the male foreskin. During sexual stimulation, by foreplay and intercourse, the clitoris enlarges by the same mechanism as does the penis, by increased blood-flow through the arteries. Such stimulation is important in helping a woman to achieve orgasm. Between the clitoris and the vaginal opening lies the opening of the urethra – the urinary opening leading from the bladder.

The hymen is a thin layer of soft skin which surrounds the vaginal opening. Its size and thickness vary greatly. Many girls and young women find the hymen becomes stretched and may be relatively non-existent by the

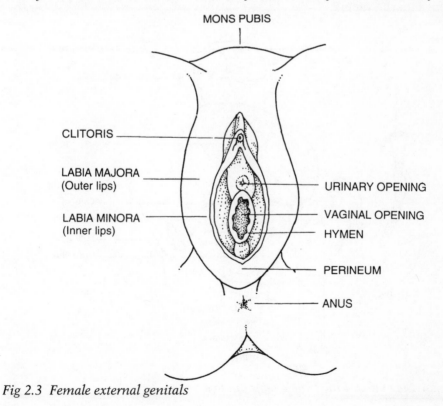

Fig 2.3 Female external genitals

time the first act of intercourse takes place. Physical activities such as gymnastics, horse riding and the use of tampons stretch the hymen. The physical state of the hymen is not always an indicator of a girl's virginity or previous sexual experience. In a small number of women, the hymen is very thick and may cause pain on penetration in the early stages of intercourse. Very rarely, the hymen may be completely closed and may need to be opened surgically to allow menstrual blood to flow at puberty.

The area of tissue between the external genitals and the anus is known as the perineum. This tissue may be damaged during childbirth. The surgical procedure of cutting the perineal tissue to enlarge the birth canal is known as episiotomy.

The external female genitals can vary quite considerably from one woman to another. The labia minora may be quite large and often of uneven size. Women should be reassured that there is a very wide range of normality.

FEMALE REPRODUCTIVE ORGANS

The female reproductive system is composed of two ovaries from each of which runs a tube known as the fallopian tube, which opens into the cavity of the uterus. The lower end of the uterus is known as the cervix and this opens into the vagina.

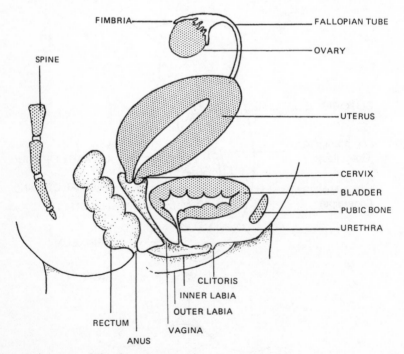

Fig 2.4 Side view of the female reproductive organs

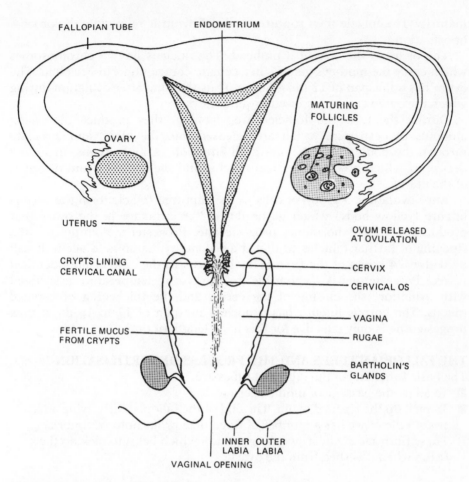

Fig 2.5 Front view of the female reproductive organs

THE OVARIES

The ovaries serve two basic functions:

■ They produce ova or egg cells, the female sex cells. In contrast to the male sperm, mature ova are not produced continuously but in a cyclical pattern. Normally only one ovum matures in each cycle.

■ The ovaries produce the female sex hormones, oestrogen and progesterone. These hormones control the menstrual cycle. They are also responsible for the development of the female secondary sex characteristics including rounding of the breasts, and the growth of pubic and axillary hair.

Ovulation and the development of the corpus luteum

The ovary contains a large number of follicles. During each cycle between three and 30 follicles prepare to ripen. Each follicle forms a small fluid-filled cavity containing the ovum. Usually only one follicle will reach full maturity. The follicle then ruptures and the ovum is released – the process of ovulation.

The ovum is the size of a pinhead. The nucleus has 23 chromosomes which carry the mother's genes – her genetic contribution to her child. The ovum has a lifespan of 12 to 24 hours. Thus the time after ovulation during which the ovum can be fertilised is quite short.

During the time the follicles are ripening, they produce increasing amounts of oestrogen, which are released into the blood and circulate through the body where they have an effect on various organs, including the cervix which produces cervical mucus, and the endometrium or lining of the uterus.

After ovulation, a group of cells in the ruptured follicle form the corpus luteum (yellow body) which is the flower-like structure in the ovary that produces a second hormone, progesterone. Progesterone suppresses the ripening of further follicles so that if a second ovulation is to occur, it will be within 24 hours of the first. (This happens in the case of non-identical twins.) Progesterone is responsible for the rise in temperature associated with ovulation, the closing of the cervix and the thickening of cervical mucus. The corpus luteum has a normal lifespan of 12 to 16 days, thus progesterone is only effective for this fixed length of time.

THE FALLOPIAN TUBES AND THE PROCESS OF FERTILISATION

The basic functions of the fallopian tubes are:

- To allow the passage of motile sperm cells.
- To pick up the ripened ovum. The end of the fallopian tube lying adjacent to the ovary has a number of finger-like projections or fimbriae. These fimbriae create a sweeping motion which helps to pick up the ovum when it is shed from the ovary.

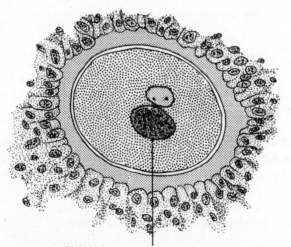

NUCLEUS containing chromosomes (mother's genes)

Fig 2.6 The ovum

■ To transport the ovum towards the cavity of the uterus. The muscular action of the tube creates peristaltic waves which transport the ovum. The microscopic hairs (cilia) lining the tubes are vital to the movement of the sperm and ovum.

Fertilisation occurs when a sperm, which has travelled up through the uterus, fuses with an ovum in the outer third of the fallopian tube. The sperm must dissolve the outer coat of the ovum by a chemical reaction, to allow penetration. Immediately one sperm has done this, a chemical barrier is formed to prevent entry of any further sperm.

The fertilised ovum or zygote receives 23 chromosomes from each parent, thus giving it a complement of 23 pairs of chromosomes – its own individual genetic structure. At this stage all the inherited characteristics are determined, for example gender, height, colour of hair and eyes.

The sex of the child is determined at the moment of conception, depending on the type of sex chromosome supplied by the sperm cell, as in Fig 2.8 (overleaf). The ovum contains 22 chromosomes plus one X sex chromosome. The sperm cell contains 22 chromosomes plus either an X or Y sex chromosome. If non-identical twins are conceived as a result of two ova being fertilised separately, they may be of like sex or different sex. If identical twins are conceived, the division occurs after the ovum has been fertilised, when the genetic complement is complete. The zygote splits to produce twins of the same sex with identical characteristics.

The rapidly developing zygote travels along the tube and after several days begins to embed in the nourishing lining of the uterus. This process,

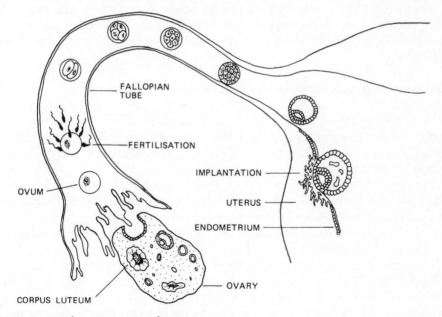

Fig 2.7 Fertilisation to implantation

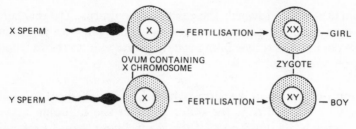

Fig 2.8 The sex of the child determined by the father

known as implantation, is complete about nine days after ovulation.

If the ovum is not fertilised it degenerates within 24 hours.

THE UTERUS

The uterus is a pear-shaped organ with a thick muscular wall. It is capable of expanding greatly during pregnancy to accommodate the growing baby. During childbirth the muscular portion must generate enough force to push the infant out through the birth canal. It must then return to its normal shape and size, to prepare for another pregnancy.

The cavity of the uterus has a lining known as the endometrium. This nourishes and protects the newly fertilised egg and assists in the formation of the placenta that will serve to nourish the infant until birth.

The endometrium, because of its vital function in sustaining pregnancy, must be in good condition and to ensure this, it is completely changed each cycle. The timing of the cyclical build-up and disintegration of the endometrium coincides with the release of an ovum. When an egg is ready to be fertilised, the endometrium will be ready to receive it. The maximal development of the endometrium coincides with the time when a fertilised egg would be expected to implant in the uterine cavity – about six days after ovulation.

Changes in the endometrium during the menstrual cycle
Menstruation
During menstruation, the thick soft endometrium which is rich in blood capillaries breaks down and is shed. The menstrual period lasts for three to seven days, the first days of bleeding being heavier since most of the tissue is shed at this time.

Biologically, menstruation occurs at the end of a cycle in which the ovum has not been fertilised. It is precipitated by a fall in the hormones oestrogen and progesterone. However, because the first day of menstruation is an easily recognisable landmark, for practical purposes it is taken as day 1 of the menstrual cycle. Day 1 is the first day of fresh red bleeding.

The length of the menstrual cycle is obtained by counting the number of days from the first day of menstruation up to, but not including, the first day of the next menstruation. Cycle lengths vary from one woman to another, and in the same woman from one cycle to another – the common pattern being around 28 days.

In anovulatory cycles, when ovulation has not occurred, the menstrual period is technically a withdrawal bleed resulting from a fall in oestrogen only, rather than a true menstrual period.

Proliferation
Following menstruation, the endometrium renews itself under oestrogen stimulation by increasing the number and size of its cells – thus becoming thicker. This phase continues until ovulation, so may be of variable length.

Secretion
Following ovulation, progesterone is produced by the corpus luteum. The endometrium has numerous mucus and sugar secreting glands which start to function under progesterone stimulation. This has a softening effect. Oestrogens continue to cause further thickening of the endometrium at this time.

If fertilisation does not occur, the corpus luteum degenerates and its hormones cease to maintain the thickened, softened endometrium. The corpus luteum has an average lifespan of 12 to 16 days, after which time it is no longer active – for this reason the secretory (post-ovulatory) phase of the cycle is a fixed length of around 14 days. At the end of this phase, menstruation recurs.

If conception takes place and the fertilised ovum successfully embeds itself in the endometrium, the developing placental tissues produce the pregnancy hormone known as human chorionic gonadotrophin (HCG) which maintains the life of the corpus luteum and hence the structure of the endometrium. Menstruation will not occur and the pregnancy will be sustained.

The menarche
The menarche is the first menstrual period a girl experiences, usually between 12 and 16 years. During the first few cycles after menarche, cycle length tends to be irregular, and in quite a high proportion of cycles ovulation does not occur. Painless menstruation normally follows an anovulatory cycle. The proportion of anovulatory cycles steadily diminishes until, as reproductive maturity is reached, almost all cycles are ovulatory. Many of the early cycles where ovulation does occur have short post-ovulatory phases, and may therefore be infertile.

It should also be noted that a girl's first ovulation may precede her first menstrual period (by around 14 days), ie it is possible for conception to occur even before a girl experiences her first period.

A young woman's cycles will normally establish themselves after several months, or a few years, into a fairly regular pattern. Cycles should only be considered irregular if they vary in length by more than seven days, for example if a woman's cycles vary from 25 to 32 days, this is still considered a regular pattern.

Adolescence can provide an excellent learning experience for a young woman first introduced to the concept of fertility awareness. By observing and recording signs of her increasing maturity, she can be helped to a better understanding of her cycles, and her physical and emotional changes. She may also be helped to gain respect for her body and her potential fertility.

From the time of the menarche, menstruation recurs in a cyclical pattern until a woman reaches 40–55 years of age, when the menopause marks the last menstrual period.

THE CERVIX

The lower portion of the uterus, known as the cervix or neck of the womb, undergoes changes during the menstrual cycle under the influence of oestrogen and progesterone. There are detectable changes in the level, position, consistency and opening of the cervix.

The cervical canal is lined with mucus-secreting membrane. In this lining, pouches or crypts are formed where sperm may collect prior to ovulation. The lower end of the cervical canal which projects into the vagina is known as the external opening or os.

The cervix has an important role to play in pregnancy and childbirth. During pregnancy it closes off completely to protect the developing baby from the non-sterile environment of the vagina. During labour and delivery, it gradually shortens and opens to allow passage of the mature baby. After delivery, it rapidly returns to its normal size, shape and function, in preparation for the next pregnancy.

Cervical mucus or cervical secretions

The cells lining the cervical canal produce the mucus secretions continuously, but the quality and quantity vary considerably throughout the cycle. The progressive changes in the characteristics of cervical mucus are under the influence of the sex hormones, oestrogen and progesterone.

During the menstrual and early pre-ovulatory phases of the cycle, when the oestrogen levels are low, the mucus is thick and sticky. It retains its shape due to its high cellular content. The mucus forms a plug, blocking the cervical canal and preventing the entry of sperm.

Approximately five or six days before ovulation, the mucus starts to flow into the vagina, under the influence of increasing oestrogens. It is first experienced as a sensation of moistness or stickiness and seen as a thick/thinner white secretion.

Approaching ovulation, the high levels of oestrogen stimulate the production of a more fluid mucus which gives a characteristic slippery, lubricative sensation at the vulva. This mucus contains an elastic gel-like substance, allowing the mucus to be stretched for several inches.

Functions of fertile mucus :

■ Provides nourishment for sperm. It has increased amounts of water, salt, sugar and amino-acids.
■ Changes the pH of the vagina. Fertile mucus is alkaline – this neutralises

Fertile mucus   Infertile mucus forming plug

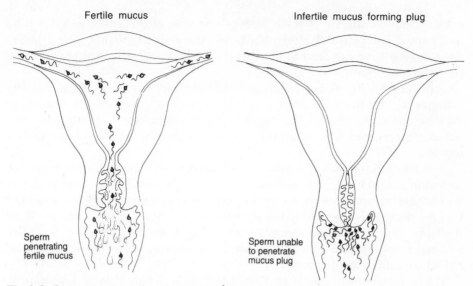

Sperm
penetrating
fertile mucus

Sperm unable
to penetrate
mucus plug

Fig 2.9 Sperm penetration in cervical mucus

the acidic vaginal secretions and provides more favourable conditions
for sperm survival.
■ Aids sperm migration.

Following ovulation, as the progesterone level rises, the mucus again
becomes thick and sticky forming a very thick plug at the cervix and preventing sperm entry. Mucus changes can be observed by women. This forms
an essential part of education in fertility awareness.

THE VAGINA
The vagina is a muscular canal leading from the cervix to the outside and is
composed of an inner layer of mucus membrane and an outer muscular
layer. The inner layer forms many folds or rugae, giving it a characteristic
ridged texture. Its opening at the vulva lies between the urethra or urinary
opening in front, and the anus behind.

Micro-organisms known as Doderleins or lactic-acid-producing bacillae
are present in the healthy vagina. These normal vaginal inhabitants dis-
courage the growth of bacteria which may enter the vagina from the
outside. Sperm cells deteriorate rapidly in the acid environment of the
vagina. They are destroyed within two to three hours, sometimes within
minutes. If fertile mucus is present, its alkaline characteristics will neutralise the acidic vagina, and allow sperm survival.

The muscular vaginal walls lie closely together, except during sexual
excitement when there is some expansion to accommodate the erect penis.
The lower end of the vagina is surrounded by a sling of voluntarily controlled muscle, which contracts to close partially the vaginal opening, and
relaxes to permit entry of the penis or allow passage of the fully developed

baby during childbirth. It is the strength or tone of this muscle that can be maintained (or restored after childbirth) through exercising. Good pelvic floor muscle tone can lead to improved bladder control, and support of the reproductive organs.

A healthy vagina is dependent on sufficient oestrogen. The vaginal lining changes during the menstrual cycle. If oestrogen levels are too low, there may be some dryness in the vagina, which could result in soreness and painful intercourse. This is a fairly common complaint among menopausal women.

The Bartholin's glands produce a colourless lubricative fluid in response to sexual stimulation. This is secreted around the vaginal opening to act as a lubricant in preparation for intercourse. Increased blood flow to vaginal tissues during sexual excitement also causes secretion of tissue fluid through the membranous vaginal walls. This 'arousal fluid' may be distinguished from cervical mucus because its texture is such that it cannot be stretched, unlike fertile mucus.

If a woman discovers an unusual vaginal discharge that is discoloured, has an offensive odour, or causes irritation, she should seek medical advice. Prompt treatment will prevent further problems. Her partner may also require treatment at the same time to prevent re-infection.

THE SEX HORMONE SYSTEM
Hormones are chemical substances which circulate in the bloodstream and control bodily functions. The reproductive cycle is under the control of sex hormones.

Cycles vary in length from 23 days or less in a short cycle, to over 35 days in a long cycle. Few women have an absolutely regular menstrual cycle, and a variation of up to seven days is perfectly normal. For convenience, we will use an average length cycle of 28 days.

Pre-ovulatory phase – controlled by FSH and oestrogen
The pituitary gland at the base of the brain secretes FSH (follicle-stimulating hormone) which, as the name implies, stimulates the ripening of follicles in the ovary. The ripening follicles produce increasing amounts of oestrogen.

Prior to ovulation as the oestrogen levels rise, certain changes take place:
- The FSH level falls, preventing the maturation of more ova.
- The cervix becomes higher and softer and the os opens slightly.
- The cervical glands produce mucus – a favourable medium for sperm.
- The endometrium becomes thicker – the proliferative phase.
- The temperature remains on the lower level.

When the oestrogens reach a certain level in the blood, the pituitary gland is stimulated to produce a sudden surge of LH (luteinising hormone) which precipitates ovulation within 36 hours. The most mature follicle ruptures and releases the ovum. This is ovulation.

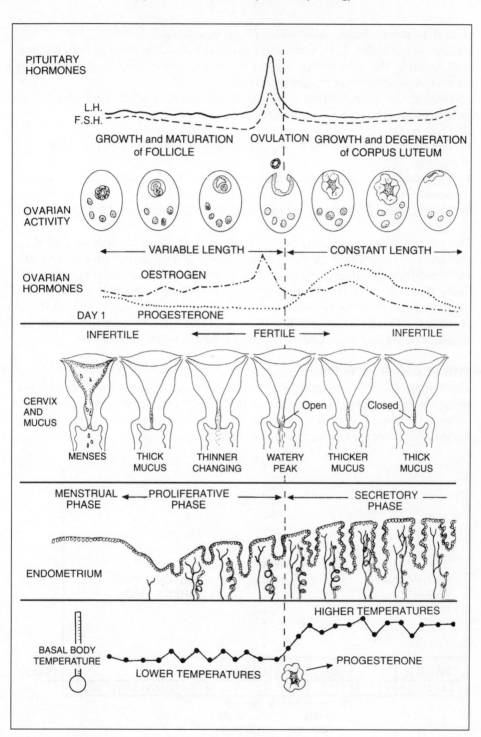

Fig 2.10 Changes during the menstrual cycle

Post-ovulatory phase – controlled by progesterone

Following ovulation LH causes the ruptured follicle to develop into the corpus luteum, the flower-like structure in the ovary which produces the second ovarian hormone – progesterone.

During the post-ovulatory phase of the cycle, under the influence of progesterone, the following changes occur :

- The cervix becomes lower and firmer and the os closes.
- The mucus becomes thick and sticky, forming an impenetrable barrier to sperm.
- The endometrium softens in preparation for the implantation of a fertilised ovum.
- The basal (waking) body temperature is raised by around 0.2°C or more.

The corpus luteum remains for around 14 days, then it shrivels and dies; the level of progesterone falls; the waking temperature drops; and the endometrium disintegrates, so completing the cycle. As the corpus luteum has a fixed lifespan, the interval between ovulation and the next menstruation is relatively constant within the range of 12 to 16 days. As menstrual cycles vary greatly in length, it follows that the interval between menstruation and ovulation must constitute the variable length of the cycle.

THE FERTILITY CYCLE

The female cycle is generally known as the menstrual cycle, menstruation being the most prominent feature of the cycle; however for purposes of fertility awareness, the cycle is often referred to as the fertility cycle, placing the emphasis on the cyclic changes of fertility.

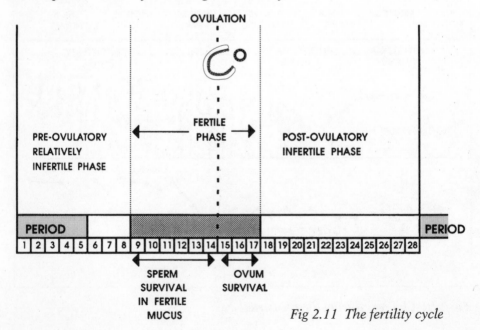

Fig 2.11 The fertility cycle

Fig 2.11 shows an average fertility cycle of 28 days. The first day of menstruation is day one of the cycle. Subsequent days are numbered up to but not including the first day of the next menstrual period. A number of infertile days follow menstruation – this is the pre-ovulatory relatively infertile phase. The fertile phase of the cycle occurs either side of ovulation. The first sign of cervical mucus heralds the onset of the fertile phase, because sperm can survive in fertile mucus awaiting ovulation. After ovulation, time must be allowed for ovum survival and the possibility of a second ovulation occurring within 24 hours. The post-ovulatory infertile phase is confirmed by a combination of temperature and mucus signs about three days after ovulation. This phase lasts until the onset of the next menstrual period. The post-ovulatory infertile phase is the most effective in avoiding pregnancy.

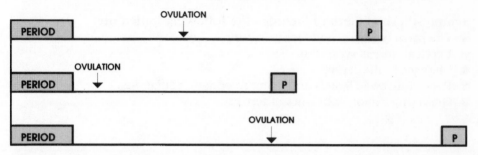

Fig 2.12 Normal length, short and long cycles. Note that the interval between ovulation and the next menstrual period remains fairly constant (around 14 days).

Fig 2.12 shows the variation in cycle length. The interval between ovulation and the next menstrual period remains fairly constant, around 14 days. Cycle lengths differ because of the variable length of the pre-ovulatory phase. In a short cycle of 21 days, ovulation will occur around day 7 and there will be no pre-ovulatory infertile days. A normal length cycle (around 28 days) will have a few pre-ovulatory relatively infertile days and a long cycle (for example 35 days) where ovulation does not occur until around day 21, will have many pre-ovulatory relatively infertile days.

A knowledge of fertility awareness allows a couple to determine the fertile and infertile phases of the cycle and thereby achieve or avoid pregnancy. Understanding the distinction between relative and absolute infertility also enables couples to adopt guidelines for avoiding pregnancy in accordance with personal circumstances.

The information contained in this book is designed to complement instruction given by a qualified fertility awareness teacher. This ensures that all the information has been adequately understood and the knowledge appropriately applied to a couple's personal circumstances. There will be many times when fertility indicators may seem obscure or external stresses may affect fertility cycles. It is vital that ongoing support is available from a recognised teacher.

It is useful to understand as much as possible about how all the indicators of fertility can be monitored – this is often called a multiple index approach. The method used throughout this book is the sympto-thermal method, in which temperature charting is combined with observation of the mucus symptom, the changes in the cervix if so wished and other minor indicators of fertility. However if a woman finds temperature taking is tiresome or unreliable because of her lifestyle, there is sufficient information here to choose a combination of indicators, for example mucus and cervix. A double check method such as this gives the most accurate information about fertility status, as there is less room for error. The essential component is flexibility. A couple need information in order to find a method that fits in with their lifestyle and can be used with confidence.

Sympto-thermal method includes the following indicators:
■ The basal (waking) body temperature.
■ Cervical mucus symptom.
■ Changes in the cervix.
■ Recording cycle length and using calendar calculations.
■ Observing minor indicators of fertility.

3. The First Indicator – Temperature

Progesterone secreted from the corpus luteum following ovulation raises the basal (waking) body temperature by around 0.2°C and maintains it at the higher level until the time of the next menstruation. This confirms that ovulation has occurred and identifies the beginning of the post-ovulatory infertile phase. Temperature readings have no value in predicting ovulation.

THERMOMETERS
There are two types of thermometer in common use:

Fertility thermometer
This mercury and glass thermometer is like a clinical thermometer, but it covers only the range from 35–39°C. This makes it easier to detect the minimal changes which occur. Special care has to be taken in using the fertility thermometer as it is very fragile. It is sensible to have two fertility thermometers available in case of breakage. (The use of a new thermometer should be recorded on the chart.)
- It must never be put in hot water.
- It should not be used if a woman suspects she has a fever.
- It should be kept away from children.
- Care must be taken when shaking it down after use. The mercury should be shaken down below 35°C the night before.

The time taken to record the temperature :
- Oral temperatures – 5 minutes
- Internal temperatures (vaginal or rectal) – 3 minutes

Fertility thermometers are not allowed on aircraft because they contain mercury.

Digital thermometer
Battery-operated digital thermometers are now chosen by many women because although they are more expensive, they are safer, being virtually unbreakable and there is no restriction on air travel. They are easy to read and the recording time is reduced. Digital thermometers give an audible bleep when the temperature has stabilised (after about one minute). This useful feature avoids the need for clock watching. Many digital thermometers also have a 'last memory recall' feature. This is particularly useful as it avoids the necessity for recording the reading immediately if this is inconvenient. It is important to follow the manufacturers' instructions and replace the battery as indicated.

RECORDING AND CHARTING
THE BASAL BODY TEMPERATURE (BBT)

1. The temperature should be taken immediately on waking before getting out of bed, drinking tea or any other activity, and at about the same time each morning. If the recording time varies by more than 1 hour, this must be noted.
2. The temperature may be taken by the mouth, vaginal or rectal routes.
   Mouth or oral route. The silvery end of the thermometer is placed under the tongue, with the lips closed for the appropriate time
   Vaginal route. The thermometer is inserted gently into the vagina.
   Rectal route. A trace of vaseline or KY jelly is smeared on the silvery end which is inserted gently into the rectum, while lying on one side with the knees drawn up.
   For accuracy, whatever route has been chosen should be followed throughout the cycle. Oral temperatures usually give satisfactory results if exact instructions are followed, but for some women internal temperatures tend to be more reliable.
3. The chart is marked with the temperature reading by a dot in the centre of the appropriate square. The dots should be joined to form a continuous graph. If one or more temperature reading is missed do not join non-consecutive dots.
   Fertility thermometer. If the mercury stops between two marks the lower reading should be recorded.
   Digital thermometer. Only record the reading to the first decimal place.
4. The thermometer should be cleaned with cotton wool and cold water.
5. A new chart is started on the first day of menstruation (fresh red bleeding). This is Day 1 of the cycle. If menstruation starts during the day, that morning's temperature should be transferred to a new chart.
6. Anything unusual should be noted on the chart, such as a cold, a late night, drinking alcohol, or any stressful situation.

INTERPRETING THE TEMPERATURE READINGS

OVULATORY CYCLES – IDENTIFYING THE TEMPERATURE SHIFT

A cycle in which ovulation has occurred is characterised by a biphasic temperature chart. The temperature remains at the lower level until the time of ovulation, when a rise or shift occurs of about 0.2°C or more. The rise usually takes place abruptly between one day and the next. The temperature remains on the higher level until just before, or at the onset of, the next period.

TO DETERMINE THE POST-OVULATORY INFERTILE PHASE

If pregnancy is to be avoided, intercourse cannot be resumed immediately the temperature shift is recorded. The ovum can be fertilised for up to 12 hours after ovulation and allowance must be made for the possibility of a second ovulation within 24 hours of the first, a rare phenomenon which occurs in twin pregnancies.

RULE OF 3 OVER 6

The post-ovulatory infertile phase begins after the third high temperature has been recorded. There must be three consecutive undisturbed high temperatures above the level of the previous six consecutive daily temperatures. The shift need only be 0.1°C but one of the three high temperatures should be at least 0.2°C above the coverline.

To identify the relevant temperatures when applying the rule of 3 over 6 (see box), a horizontal coverline is drawn on the line immediately above the highest of the low temperatures. A vertical line is then drawn, forming a cross on the chart between the two days when the temperature shift from the lower to the higher phase occurred. This is illustrated in Fig 3.1 with the three higher temperatures in the upper right quadrant and the previous six in the lower left quadrant. As soon as the third high temperature has been recorded, intercourse can be resumed and the rest of the cycle will be infertile.

The 3 over 6 rule is very efficient and simple to use and for this reason is the method adopted here for identifying the post-ovulatory infertile phase for women of normal fertility.

The coverline technique helps to avoid errors of interpretation when there is any doubt about the accuracy of the six low temperatures, for example when there is a particularly disturbed chart, or in special circum-

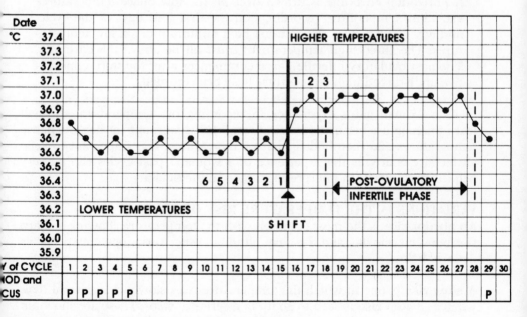

Fig 3.1 Biphasic chart showing rule of 3 over 6

35

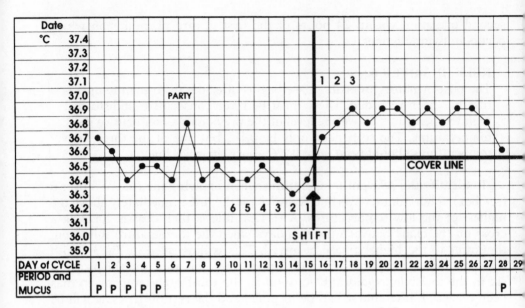

Fig 3.2 Use of a coverline to determine the temperature shift

stances such as during breast-feeding, post-pill or during the pre-menopause.

COVERLINE TECHNIQUE

A horizontal coverline is drawn over all the low phase temperatures excluding temperature recordings on the first four days of the cycle, and any disturbances. There must be a minimum of six low temperatures. The three high temperatures must all be above the coverline. The post-ovulatory infertile phase commences after the third consecutive undisturbed high temperature has been recorded.

As a woman gains experience in recording her temperature, she will learn to recognise her usual coverline and the usual range for her low phase temperatures and then higher phase temperatures. It is important to keep all fertility charts as the experience of a woman's past cycles can be very helpful, particularly in interpreting a more difficult chart.

VARIATIONS IN THE TEMPERATURE RISE OR SHIFT

An abrupt rise is the most common with the temperature showing a sharp rise between one day and the next, although other variations may occur as detailed below.

A slow rise is one in which the temperature rises slowly over several days whereas a **step rise** is seen to go up in a series of steps. These are shown in Fig 3.3 and may easily be interpreted using the rule of 3 over 6.

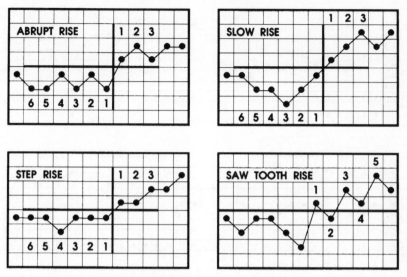

Fig 3.3 Variations in the temperature shift

A saw tooth rise goes through a series of peaks and troughs and although very rare is more difficult to interpret – experienced help is needed. By drawing a coverline, identify the beginning of the rise. The post-ovulatory infertile phase begins after the fifth temperature has been recorded as in Fig 3.3.

VARIATIONS IN SHIFT DAY

Cycle lengths will vary considerably, but as the temperature shift occurs 12–16 days before the next period it will be apparent that it will occur earlier in shorter cycles and later in longer cycles as demonstrated in Fig 3.4 (overleaf). The length of the pre-ovulatory infertile phase will vary accordingly but the post-ovulatory infertile phase will remain constant.

A SPIKE

A temperature spike is defined as a single recording which is 0.2°C or more above its immediate neighbours as in Fig 3.5 (overleaf). A spike may result from a disturbance caused by drinking alcohol, a late night, oversleeping, minor illness or stress. Sometimes there may be no obvious cause for a spike. When interpreting the chart it is often helpful to circle the spike so that the disturbance is easily recognised.

One temperature spike may safely be ignored when determining the six temperatures on the lower level, but where possible there should be an explanation for the temperature disturbance. If more than one spike is present, then it is advisable to wait a further few days until the position becomes clear again. If a disturbance affects one of the three higher temperatures, it is advisable to wait for a fourth high temperature to ensure infertility.

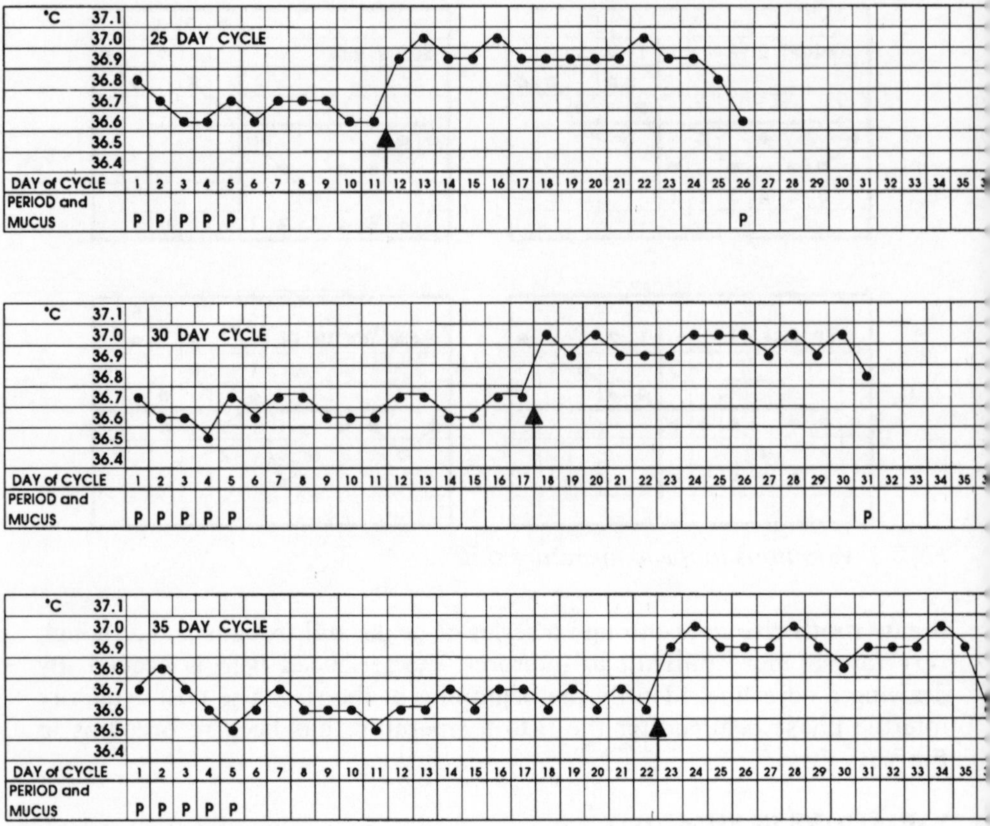

Fig 3.4 Variations in shift day. Arrows show thermal shift.

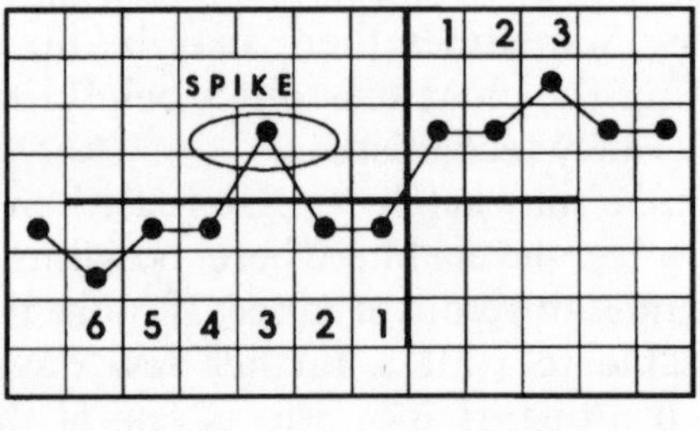

Fig 3.5 Disturbance producing a spike

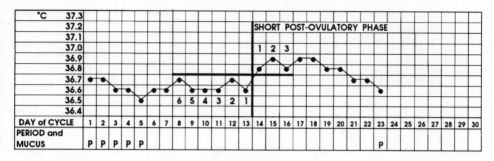

Fig 3.6 Biphasic chart with short post-ovulatory phase

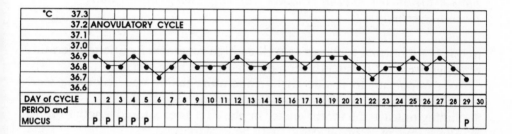

Fig 3.7 Monophasic chart indicating anovulatory cycle. Note absence of temperature shift.

SHORT POST-OVULATORY PHASE

Some women will experience cycles with a shortened post-ovulatory phase, as in Fig 3.6. If the post-ovulatory or luteal phase lasts less than nine days, the cycle will be infertile as there is insufficient time for implantation to take place. This can only be seen retrospectively. Short luteal phases may be observed during times of stress or during special circumstances. This is of particular significance for couples planning pregnancy.

ANOVULATORY CYCLES

In a small proportion of cycles, ovulation does not occur. Anovulatory cycles are characterised by a monophasic chart, that is the temperature readings remain on one level throughout the cycle as shown in Fig 3.7. This may be contrasted with the distinct biphasic pattern demonstrated by the ovulatory cycle in Fig 3.6. Anovulatory cycles are more common at the extremes of the fertile life, adolescence and the pre-menopause. They may also occur after childbirth, and after coming off the contraceptive pill.

FAULTY RECORDING TECHNIQUE

A very erratic temperature chart may indicate faulty recording technique as in Fig 3.8 (overleaf). It differs from a chart affected by illness, by showing

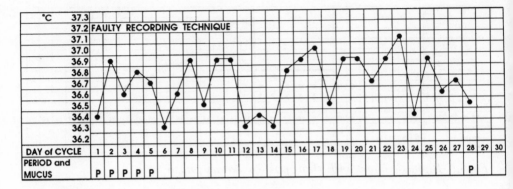

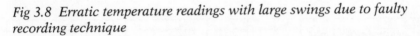

Fig 3.8 Erratic temperature readings with large swings due to faulty recording technique

frequent subnormal readings as well as high readings. Erratic temperature readings are most frequently seen during the learning phase.

It is important to ensure that temperature-taking and recording techniques are thoroughly understood. Common errors include :

■ Failing to leave the thermometer in place for the required length of time.
■ Alterations in recording time (with no explanation).
■ Alterations in route mid-cycle.
■ Change of thermometer mid-cycle.
■ Possible battery failure – digital thermometer.
■ Failing to shake the mercury down properly – fertility thermometer.

If the temperature is being taken orally, it may be wise to change to the vaginal or rectal route at the beginning of the next cycle, if this is acceptable. This tends to give a more stable pattern which is easier to interpret.

4. The Second Indicator – Cervical Mucus

During the menstrual cycle changes take place in the mucus produced by the glands or crypts in the cervix. These changes have been observed and their significance understood over the centuries by certain tribes in Africa and peoples in Southern Asia. Many women in western countries notice the mucus symptom, but are unaware of its significance.

> **BECKY:** *Becky is an art student. For some months she had been concerned about a discharge that seemed to come every few weeks and last four or five days. When she heard a speaker on 'Fertility Awareness' at a college meeting she heaved a sigh of relief. The discharge that she had connected with infection and possible lack of hygiene was not only normal but was her body's way of offering her a very obvious sign about the state of her fertility.*

RECOGNITION OF CERVICAL MUCUS

Cervical mucus can be recognised by sensation, by appearance and by testing with the finger.

SENSATION
Sensation is very important and often the most difficult to learn. Throughout the day the presence or absence of mucus will be recognised by the sensation at the vulva, the way the beginning of a period is noticed. The sensation may be a distinct feeling of dryness, of dampness or moistness, stickiness, wetness or slipperiness.

APPEARANCE
Soft white toilet tissue should be used to blot or wipe the vulva. There may be dampness only on the tissue resulting from the moistness associated with the vagina. This moistness soaks into the tissue and any cervical mucus will appear raised as a blob on the tissue.

The colour should be noted. It may be white, creamy, opaque, or transparent. Mucus is often noticed on underclothing, where it will have dried slightly causing some alteration in its characteristics.

FINGER TESTING
A finger-tip can be lightly applied to the mucus on the tissue and then pulled gently away to test its capacity to stretch. It may feel sticky and

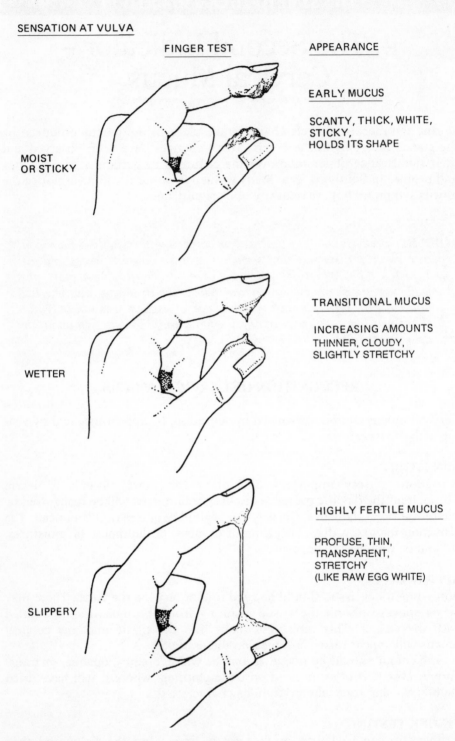

SENSATION AT VULVA

FINGER TEST

APPEARANCE

EARLY MUCUS

SCANTY, THICK, WHITE, STICKY, HOLDS ITS SHAPE

MOIST OR STICKY

TRANSITIONAL MUCUS

INCREASING AMOUNTS THINNER, CLOUDY, SLIGHTLY STRETCHY

WETTER

HIGHLY FERTILE MUCUS

PROFUSE, THIN, TRANSPARENT, STRETCHY (LIKE RAW EGG WHITE)

SLIPPERY

Fig 4.1 Characteristics of cervical mucus

break easily, or it may feel smoother and slippery like raw egg white and stretch between the thumb and first finger, from a little up to several centimetres before it breaks. This stretchiness is described as the Spinnbarkeit or Spinn effect, and shows that the mucus is highly fertile.

CHANGES IN CERVICAL MUCUS DURING THE FERTILITY CYCLE

PRE-OVULATORY RELATIVELY INFERTILE PHASE
Following the menstrual period there may be several dry days. These days may be absent in short cycles and numerous in long cycles. A feeling of dryness or a positive sensation of nothingness at the vulva will be experienced. There will be no visible mucus.

THE FERTILE PHASE
As the oestrogen levels rise, cervical mucus will be felt at the vulva. At first it will give a sensation of moistness or stickiness and will appear in scant amounts – white or creamy coloured. On finger-testing, the mucus will hold its shape and break easily.

The mucus goes through a transitional phase where increasing amounts of cloudy mucus secretion may be observed. It may be slightly stretchy on finger testing, producing a wetter sensation at the vulva.

As the oestrogen levels continue to rise with approaching ovulation, the mucus will become more profuse, and there may be up to a tenfold increase in volume. It will give a sensation of lubrication or slipperiness at the vulva. The appearance will be similar to that of raw egg white, thin, watery and transparent. On finger-testing, this highly fertile mucus may stretch for several centimetres before it breaks.

Fertile mucus maintains the life of sperm, nourishes it and allows it to pass freely through the cervix. In fertile mucus, sperm may live for up to three days, in rare circumstances for five days or even longer.

PEAK DAY
Peak day denotes the LAST day on which this highly fertile-type slippery, transparent, stretchy mucus is either seen or felt.

GUIDELINES FOR ACHIEVING PREGNANCY – USING MUCUS SYMPTOM ONLY
■ Couples wishing to achieve pregnancy should have intercourse on any day when highly fertile-type mucus is present.
■ Frequently the day of maximum amount of highly fertile mucus precedes peak day by one or two days. Peak day and the two days preceding peak are the days of maximum fertility.

POST-OVULATORY COMPLETELY INFERTILE PHASE
During the post-ovulatory phase, following peak day the slippery sensation

is lost and there will be a relatively abrupt return to stickiness or dryness again. This reflects the presence of progesterone, which thickens the mucus again forming a plug at the cervix that acts as an impenetrable barrier to sperm.

The amount and quality of mucus will vary from woman to woman and also from one cycle to the next. A woman should be alert to any changes in sensation and to even relatively small amounts of mucus.

If a woman is finding difficulty detecting mucus externally, it is often recognised more easily after exercise or a bowel movement. It may also help to use the Kegel exercise (see page 51) or a slight bearing down action to expel any mucus.

DETECTION OF MUCUS IN THE FIRST CYCLE OF CHARTING

During the first cycle of the learning phase, it is advisable to abstain from intercourse completely until the post-ovulatory infertile phase has been confirmed in conjunction with an NFP teacher. This allows time for a woman to familiarise herself with both the change from dryness as the mucus first appears and the progressive changes in her mucus pattern, without possible confusion from either seminal or arousal fluids.

GUIDELINES FOR AVOIDING PREGNANCY – USING MUCUS SYMPTOM ONLY

Pre-ovulatory relatively infertile phase

■ Dry days following the period are relatively infertile. Any change from the sensation of true dryness or any visible mucus warns of approaching fertility and should be regarded as fertile.

■ Intercourse should be restricted to evenings to allow time for observation of mucus symptom during the day.

■ It is unwise to have intercourse on consecutive evenings to avoid confusion between cervical mucus and seminal fluid.

■ Safe on alternate dry evenings.

Post-ovulatory infertile phase

■ If a woman is relying on the mucus symptom alone, the post-ovulatory infertile phase starts on the fourth evening past peak day. (This interval allows for the fact that peak day does not coincide precisely with the day of ovulation. It allows for the life of the ovum and makes provision for a second ovulation.)

OVULATION OR MUCUS METHOD (BILLINGS METHOD)

Drs John and Evelyn Billings have developed earlier scientific knowledge of mucus changes into a practical method where, by observation of mucus signs alone, a woman can be aware of her natural fertility and use the

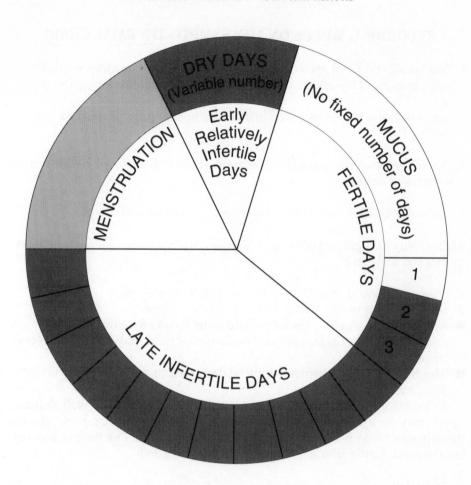

Fig 4.2 The mucus pattern of fertility and infertility (Billings)

knowledge to achieve or avoid pregnancy. They have their own method of charting and rules. This is commonly known as the Billings method, and is used by many people throughout the world. It is the method of choice in many of the developing countries.

OVULATION METHOD (CREIGHTON MODEL)

Professor Thomas Hilgers in the USA has devised a scoring system, known as the Creighton model, to grade different types of mucus according to characteristics of sensation, colour and consistency. This is similar to the scoring system used in fertility clinics. Many women use this method effectively, relying on mucus signs alone. It requires a full programme of instruction by a qualified teacher of the method.

RECORDING MUCUS ON THE SYMPTO-THERMAL CHART

1. Mucus should be observed throughout the day and the chart marked each evening. This allows changes to become apparent during the day.

2. Each day of a period or blood loss, including spotting, is marked with a **P**.

3. Each day when there is a dry sensation at the vulva and no visible mucus is marked with a **D**.

4. Each day of sticky white/creamy mucus is marked with an **M**.

5. Each day of highly fertile wet or slippery, transparent, stretchy mucus is marked with an **F**.

6. A woman should describe the mucus in her own words.
   - **Sensation**: eg moist, sticky, wet, lubricative, slippery.
   - **Appearance** or colour on soft, white toilet tissue, for example white, creamy, cloudy, or transparent. Fertile-type mucus may be slightly blood-tinged.
   - **The finger test**: consistency may be described as sticky, thready or stretchy.

   In practice the characteristic mucus changes may not be well defined. There may be a combination of two types of mucus, for example cloudy, thready mucus with some transparent stretchy mucus. The mucus possessing the more fertile characteristics should be recorded.

7. Peak day

This is marked with a cross through the last **F**. Remember that peak day denotes the LAST day of highly fertile mucus (symbolised by an **F**), ie last day when slippery, transparent, stretchy mucus is present. This is not necessarily the day of the most profuse mucus. Peak day will only be known in retrospect. On the day following peak, there will be a change to the thick, white, sticky mucus again, or to dryness.

8. Intercourse

Each act of intercourse is marked with an **I** or by circling the appropriate day. If avoiding pregnancy, the significant acts to be recorded are the last intercourse before and the first intercourse after the fertile phase.

9. Any additional signs relevant to fertility awareness can be recorded, for example one-sided abdominal pain or mood variations including increased libido.

DAY of CYCLE	1	2	3	4	5	6	7	8	9	10	11	12	13	14	15	16	17	18	19	20	21	22	23	24	25	26	27	28	29	30
PERIOD and MUCUS	P	P	P	P	P	D	D	D																					P	
						DRY - NOTHING	DRY - NOTHING	DRY - NOTHING																						

Fig 4.3. *The period and dry days – 28 day cycle. The first day of menstruation (fresh red bleeding) is the first day of the cycle. A variable number of dry days marked D may follow the period.*

DAY of CYCLE	1	2	3	4	5	6	7	8	9	10	11	12	13	14	15	16	17	18	19	20	21	22	23	24	25	26	27	28	29	30
PERIOD and MUCUS	P	P	P	P	P	M	M																			P				
						MOIST-WHITE-STICKY	MOIST-WHITE-STICKY																							

Fig 4.4 *Onset of mucus immediately after the period – 25 day cycle. Days marked M indicate the presence of mucus and the absence of pre-ovulatory dry days. This is more common in short cycles.*

DAY of CYCLE	1	2	3	4	5	6	7	8	9	10	11	12	13	14	15	16	17	18	19	20	21	22	23	24	25	26	27	28	29	30
PERIOD and MUCUS	P	P	P	P	P	D	D	M	M	M																		P		
								MOIST SENSATION	MOIST-WHITE-STICKY	STICKY - CLOUDY																				

Fig 4.5 *Onset of mucus after dry days – 27 day cycle. Dry days marked D are followed by the onset of mucus on day 8. It is important to recognise the change in sensation at the vulva from true dryness to moistness. Days of moist or sticky sensation or appearance of sticky white or cloudy mucus are marked with an M and described appropriately.*

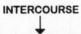

INTERCOURSE

DAY of CYCLE	1	2	3	4	5	6	⑦	8	9	10	11	12	13	14	15	16	17	18	19	20	21	22	23	24	25	26	27	28	29	30
PERIOD and MUCUS	P	P	P	P	P	D	D	M	D	D																				P

Fig 4.6 Recording a wet day the day after intercourse in the pre-ovulatory phase. During the learning phase the day after intercourse is marked as wet (M) because of the difficulty in distinguishing mucus from seminal fluid.
Note: *Intercourse during the early dry days is unlikely to lead to pregnancy, although there is always some risk in the pre-ovulatory phase.*

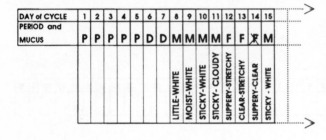

Fig 4.7a Mucus pattern approaching peak day. Any days of highly fertile clear stretchy mucus giving a wet or slippery sensation are marked with an F. The last F day is peak day and is marked with a cross through the F.

Fig 4.7b Peak day and the change after peak. After peak day, there is an abrupt change to sticky mucus or dryness. If relying on mucus symptom alone, four days marked 1,2,3,4, must elapse before intercourse can be resumed on the evening of the fourth day.

DAY of CYCLE	1	2	3	4	5	6	7	8	9	10	11	12	13	14	15	16	17	⑱	19	20	21	22	23	24	25	26	27	28	29	30
																1	2	3	4											
PERIOD and MUCUS	P	P	P	P	P	D	D	M	M	M	M	F	F	✗	M	M	M	D	D	D	D	D	D	D	D	D	D	D	D	P

Fig 4.7c Mucus changes throughout the cycle. Complete cycle showing typical pattern of menstruation, pre-ovulatory dry days, mucus days with increasingly fertile characteristics approaching peak day, the abrupt change back to less fertile characteristics, the count of four after peak day and post-ovulatory dry days.

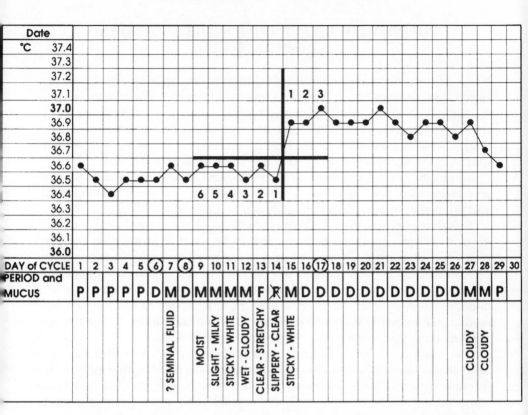

Fig 4.8 Combining the temperature and mucus recordings. This is a 28 day cycle with a five day period. The first mucus is recognised on day 9 as a moist sensation. Peak day is day 14 (the last F day), and the temperature shift is observed on day 15. The mucus on days 27 and 28 is related to hormonal fluctuations prior to the next period. Any mucus observed during the post-ovulatory infertile phase can be disregarded.

The couple are using fertility awareness to avoid pregnancy. They had intercourse on alternate dry evenings 6 and 8 and then abstained from the onset of the mucus symptom until the post-ovulatory infertile phase was confirmed by the third high temperature past peak day on day 17. The rest of the cycle was then available for unrestricted intercourse.

WHERE DOUBLE CHECK OF TEMPERATURE AND MUCUS IS USED:
■ The beginning of the fertile phase is recognised by the first mucus symptom.
■ The post-ovulatory infertile phase starts after the third high temperature has been recorded provided all three temperatures are past the peak mucus day.

COPING WITH DIFFICULTIES IN DISTINGUISHING CERVICAL MUCUS

Some women may have considerable difficulty determining changes in sensation, or distinguishing cervical mucus changes; others may have a continuous discharge confusing the picture. Women in developing countries apparently have no difficulty distinguishing mucus externally. They tend to wear loose clothes, often with no underwear, and so the sensation of mucus at the vulva is experienced and is easily interpreted.

To ensure normal sensation at the vulva, and to keep the area cool, pants should be all-cotton, as they are more absorbent and cooler. Nylon tights and other synthetic underclothing should be avoided.

It is essential to maintain normal hygiene of the genital area but baby soap, or simple, non-allergic soap should be used. Perfumed or coloured soaps and even bath oils or salts may cause minor allergic reactions of the delicate skin at the vulva. Some women may be allergic to certain washing powders, or to fabric softeners. Talcum powder, vaginal deodorants and douches should never be used. These products may neutralise the acid medium and destroy the normal flora inhabiting the vagina, hence the normal self-cleansing mechanism of the vagina will be lost.

The way in which a woman deals with her menstrual bleeding may also affect her ability to distinguish mucus. It is advisable not to use internal tampons when the menstrual flow is very light, as they may cause some drying of the vagina, and the normal flora of the vagina may be removed along with the tampon. This may cause a reactive discharge from the vaginal walls.

Finally, it has been found that overwork and stress may also predispose to vaginal discharges. Good general health and dietary habits will help to maintain the normal health of the vagina. An alteration to various practices of hygiene or clothing, or attention to diet and general health and fitness, may be all that is necessary to reduce minor vaginal discharges so that cervical mucus is more easily identified.

Some women may not experience true dry days but instead will experience a continuous pattern of discharge with more highly fertile mucus characteristics becoming apparent for a few days. These women may find the 'glass of water test' a useful means of determining whether the secretion is of cervical or vaginal origin.

GLASS OF WATER TEST
Insert two fingers containing the secretion to be tested into a glass of water. Cervical mucus is insoluble and will form a blob, falling to the bottom of the glass. Vaginal secretions will disperse.

THE KEGEL EXERCISE –
AS AN AID TO FERTILITY AWARENESS

This simple exercise is performed by alternately contracting and relaxing the pelvic floor muscles (around the entrance to the vagina).

To help identify these muscles, a woman can practise by using them to stop a flow of urine mid-stream. A further useful exercise is to insert one or two fingers into the vagina, then try to contract the muscles strongly, to grip the fingers, then relax.

The Kegel exercise forms the basis of antenatal exercises designed to improve pelvic tone in preparation for childbirth. It is also used as part of the postnatal exercise programme to strengthen the pelvic floor muscles which have been subjected to considerable stress during pregnancy and childbirth. The exercise can be a valuable aid to fertility awareness.

The Kegel exercise will help to increase awareness of the sensation at the vulva, when performed periodically during the normal course of the day. The way in which the labia separate is most important in determining the presence or absence of cervical mucus.

The pelvic floor muscles are first contracted, then relaxed. If there is no mucus present, the labia feel dry, giving a positive sensation of 'nothingness'. If sticky mucus is present, the inner labia separate in a sticky fashion and if slippery lubricative mucus is present, the labia slide smoothly away from one another.

If the Kegel exercise is performed effectively, then with experience, a woman will be able to identify true dryness or the presence of mucus on the day following intercourse. This experience is invaluable in the pre-ovulatory phase of the cycle, as it overrides the need for restricting intercourse to alternate evenings.

As an added bonus, a woman who has good control of her pelvic floor muscles may find increased pleasure during lovemaking. With her ability to contract these muscles strongly as desired, a woman may increase her partner's pleasure, and achieve her own orgasm more easily.

5. Factors Affecting the Menstrual Cycle

DISTURBANCES AFFECTING THE SYMPTO-THERMAL CHART

Any disturbance or change from normal routine must be noted on the sympto-thermal chart so that the effect on the cycle can be ascertained.

A disturbed night's sleep can affect the following morning's temperature reading but provided the temperature is taken after at least 3 hours rest in bed, the recording should be accurate. A late night and alcohol may affect the temperature, giving a false high or low reading, depending on the individual.

Rising later in the morning may affect the temperature. Our body clock is based on a circadian rhythm ie over 24 hours. It is generally noted that the basal (waking) body temperature rises by about 0.1°C per hour, so that taking the temperature at 9 am instead of the usual 7 am will increase it by 0.2°C. Likewise, if the temperature is taken much earlier than usual it will be correspondingly lower.

The inclusion of the days of the week in addition to the dates can be very helpful when looking at the occurrence of disturbances. The temperature may be higher at weekends due to lying in bed, alcohol, etc. either producing temperature spikes, or alternatively, falsely high readings on two or more consecutive days. It is vital to mark disturbances clearly on the chart.

Holidays and travel may delay or suppress ovulation. Air travel which involves crossing time-zones and upsets the body's natural rhythm is likely to make reliable temperature recordings impossible. It may take about a week for the body to adapt to such changes. A holiday proved to be the problem in the following case.

AMANDA AND STEPHEN: 'I really don't want to be sterilised,' said Amanda after her third child. 'I am only 26 and we may want another baby in a year or two.'

Amanda suffered from allergies; barrier methods were out, the coil had caused her severe backache and very heavy periods, and she felt unwell on the pill. She and Stephen went to a class to learn about natural methods. Amanda's cycles were regular, mucus signs were recognised in the first month and her temperature charts were classical.

Then came the holiday of a lifetime on a Greek Island. Amanda accidentally left her thermometer and charts at home. 'Never mind', she told Stephen, 'We can rely on mucus signs.' Amanda discovered she was pregnant three weeks later. Relying solely on mucus signs was not so easy for her when half the day was spent in the sea. Amanda told her friends about natural methods, but her enthusiasm somehow lacked conviction!

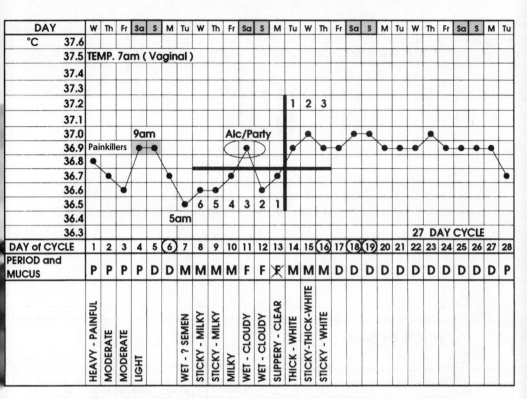

DAY		W	Th	Fr	Sa	S	M	Tu	W	Th	Fr	Sa	S	M	Tu	W	Th	Fr	Sa	S	M	Tu	W	Th	Fr	Sa	S	M	Tu
°C	37.6																												
	37.5	TEMP. 7am (Vaginal)																											
	37.4																												
	37.3																												
	37.2												1	2	3														
	37.1																												
	37.0				9am					Alc/Party																			
	36.9	Painkillers																											
	36.8																												
	36.7																												
	36.6																												
	36.5								6	5	4	3	2	1															
	36.4					5am																							
	36.3																					27 DAY CYCLE							
DAY of CYCLE		1	2	3	4	5	(6)	7	8	9	10	11	12	13	14	15	(16)	17	(18)	(19)	20	21	22	23	24	25	26	27	28
PERIOD and MUCUS		P	P	P	P	D	D	M	M	M	M	F	F	✗	M	M	M	D	D	D	D	D	D	D	D	D	D	D	P

Fig 5.1 Effect of common disturbances. This 27 day cycle has a temperature shift on day 14. Peak mucus day is on day 13. The post-ovulatory infertile phase starts on day 16 after the third high temperature past peak day. Note the disturbance to the temperature caused by alcohol, changes in recording time and the weekend days 4 and 5.

THE POSSIBLE EFFECTS OF STRESS ON THE CYCLE

Women using natural family planning should be aware of the effect stress may have on the cycle. It may affect hormonal control and ovarian function to varying degrees, resulting in either a delayed ovulation or the complete suppression of ovulation.

If the stress occurs during the pre-ovulatory phase, then the mucus pattern may be interrupted. There may be a return to dryness, as illustrated in Fig 5.2 (overleaf). Ovulation will be delayed either until the stress is over or the body adapts to it. Ovarian function will then return to normal and the mucus pattern will show the characteristic build-up to peak.

Some women may experience more than one peak day when under stress, resulting in double or multiple peaks. This is seen as a build-up to peak day followed by a return to dryness or sticky mucus days, then a further episode of clear stretchy mucus several days later. If a double peak

DAY of CYCLE	1	2	3	4	5	6	⑦	8	9	10	11	12	13	14	15	16	17	18	19	20	㉑	22	23	24	25	26	27	28	29	30	31	32	33	34
PERIOD and MUCUS																		1	2	3	4													
	P	P	P	P	P	D	D	M	M	M	D	D	M	M	F	F	✗	M	D	D	D	D	D	D	D	D	D	D	D	D	P			

Mucus descriptions: day 8 MOIST - ONLY; day 9 STICKY - WHITE; day 10 STICKY - WHITE; day 13 MOIST - WHITE; day 14 STICKY - WHITE; day 15 WET - CLOUDY; day 16 TRANSPARENT - SPINN; day 17 SLIPPERY - TRANSPARENT; day 18 STICKY - WHITE.

Fig 5.2 Interrupted mucus pattern as a result of stress. Once the mucus symptom has started any return to dryness (days 11 and 12) should be considered fertile. The fertile phase extends from days 8 to 20 inclusive.

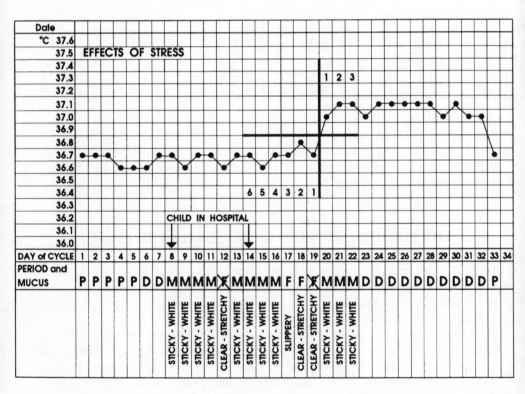

Fig 5.3 Double peak caused by stress. Note: *The first peak day is on day 12 , but the temperature shift is delayed until after the second peak on day 19. The fertile phase extends from days 8 to 21 inclusive.*

occurs, the temperature shift will be delayed until after the second peak has been observed.

When multiple peaks occur due to several unsuccessful attempts at ovulation, the temperature shift will be delayed until after the final 'true' peak. The temperature shift is the most reliable means of confirming that ovulation has occurred. To avoid making errors in chart interpretation, it is vital to correlate temperature readings with mucus changes. Surprise pregnancies have occurred when couples tire of waiting for the temperature shift and presume a cycle to be infertile.

If the stress is very severe, for example a bereavement or major accident, ovulation may be completely suppressed. The periods may also stop in some cases. The basic infertile pattern may be one of dryness throughout, or of unchanging mucus characteristics. There may be mucus changes associated with fluctuating hormone levels, but the temperature will remain on one level until the next period, indicating an anovulatory cycle. Ovulation may be delayed by stress for many months in extreme circumstances, for example when there has been severe weight loss as in anorexia nervosa.

THE EFFECT OF ILLNESS AND MEDICATION ON THE CYCLE

Feverish illness will cause a rise in temperature (pyrexia). However this rise will be much higher than the rise which occurs at the time of ovulation and so should not cause confusion in interpreting the temperature chart. If pyrexia occurs in the pre-ovulatory phase and is over before ovulation, the temperature will return to the low level and the ovulation shift will be observed later, as in Fig 5.4. However if the pyrexia occurs around the time of ovulation, the temperature may be seen to fall to the level of the higher phase temperatures, indicating that the ovulation shift occurred during the illness, as in Fig 5.5. The woman's usual coverline can be used to help determine the position in her cycle. Mucus changes will also act as a double check where there is any disturbance to the temperature readings.

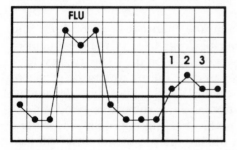

Fig 5.4 Pyrexia in the pre-ovulatory phase

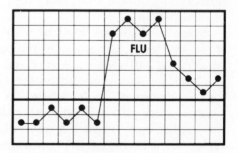

Fig 5.5 Pyrexia around the time of ovulation

CERVICAL ECTROPIAN (OR EROSION)

A cervical ectropian, or erosion, occurs when the lining of the cervical canal grows over the lip of the cervix. When seen through a speculum it appears as a red, raw area on the cervix, which is normally pinkish-coloured. There is an increased incidence of cervical ectropian as a response to oestrogen following childbirth, and also as a side effect of the contraceptive pill.

The cells of the ectropian may produce a continuous discharge. With experience, a woman will generally learn to distinguish this from her fertile mucus pattern. The ectropian may cause a characteristic unchanging mucus pattern throughout the cycle. The onset and build-up of fertile mucus will be recognised as being significantly different. If the discharge is excessive, it may cause a problem, and the affected area can be treated using cryosurgery (freezing), or laser therapy. Following such treatment, there may be a heavy, thick discharge for about two weeks before the number of mucus days returns to normal. In most women, the cervical ectropian causes no symptoms and is best left alone.

MEDICATION

Some drugs will affect the menstrual cycle and cause irregularities in the cycle length, the mucus pattern or the temperature. If drugs are prescribed to treat infections, the disturbance may be caused as much by the infection and the stress it imposes on the body as by the medication. Any infection is likely to be accompanied by a pyrexia (fever), thus disturbing the temperature pattern.

Some analgesics (painkillers), such as aspirin and paracetamol, also act to reduce pyrexia. These drugs may therefore produce a lower than normal temperature reading.

The cervical mucus pattern may be disturbed by antibiotics. Some women develop thrush, a yeast infection due to the alteration of the normal vaginal medium after a course of antibiotics.

Antihistamine drugs dry up excessive secretions from mucus membranes. As the cervix is lined by mucus membrane, the drying effect may disrupt cervical secretion. The production of cervical mucus may also be impaired by anti-inflammatory drugs, such as those used in the treatment of rheumatism.

Some medications used to treat migraine, nausea, and vomiting and travel sickness; chemotherapy, the powerful drugs used in the treatment of cancer; and cortisone may also cause irregularities in the menstrual cycle.

Oestrogen and progestogen therapy, used in the treatment of gynaecological disorders, will affect the quality and quantity of mucus. Contraceptive pills will suppress ovulation and the subjective symptoms of the fertility cycle, in such a way as to make charting impossible. Hormone replacement therapy (HRT) prescribed during the pre-menopause will also affect the sympto-thermal chart.

The following is a checklist of factors which may affect the sympto-thermal chart:

- Alcohol
- Late night
- Disturbed night
- Oversleeping
- Holidays
- Travel
- Time zones
- Shift work
- Stress
- Illness
- Gynaecological disorders
- Medication

Fertility awareness enables a woman to be more in tune with her body's natural changes and she will be very quickly alerted to any abnormalities which may affect her sexual health.

6. The Third Indicator – Cervix

CHANGES IN THE CERVIX

To use the sympto-thermal method effectively, it is not essential to check the cervix. Temperature and mucus observations give a woman adequate information about her state of fertility. However, some women find that monitoring changes directly at the cervix gives additional supportive information. In special circumstances, such as during breast-feeding and the pre-menopause, it can give valuable early warning signs of approaching fertility.

Changes in the cervix are due to the effect of the hormones oestrogen and progesterone. During the infertile phases of the cycle, the cervix is low in the vagina, and easily within reach of the fingertip. It appears to be long and may be off-centre, tilted, to lie against the vaginal wall. It will feel firm, like the tip of a nose. The cervical opening (os) will be closed, giving the sensation of a dimple to the touch, and it will feel dry.

As ovulation approaches, the rising oestrogen levels cause the cervix to rise higher in the vagina. It appears shorter, straighter and more centrally positioned in the vagina. It may be difficult to reach. It will feel softer, more like the texture of the lower lip. The cervix relaxes slightly, allowing the os to open enough to admit the finger-tip. It will feel wet and flowing with mucus.

The changes in the cervix take place over an interval of around 10 days. Approximately six days before the shift in temperature the cervix will begin to show fertile characteristics. Following ovulation, the cervix returns to its infertile state within 24–48 hours.

GUIDELINES FOR INTERPRETING CERVICAL SIGNS:
■ A low, long, tilted, firm, closed, dry cervix indicates infertility.
■ A high, short, straight, soft, open, wet cervix indicates fertility.

To conceive, intercourse should coincide with the signs of maximum fertility.
To avoid pregnancy, intercourse should be avoided from the onset of fertile signs until the third evening of the post-ovulatory infertile cervix.
Cervical signs alone should not be relied upon as a means of avoiding pregnancy.

The subtle changes in level, position, consistency and dilatation of the cervix occur gradually and may seem confusing at first, but with experience a woman will be able to recognise at least one of the characteristics which will give clear indication of her state of fertility.

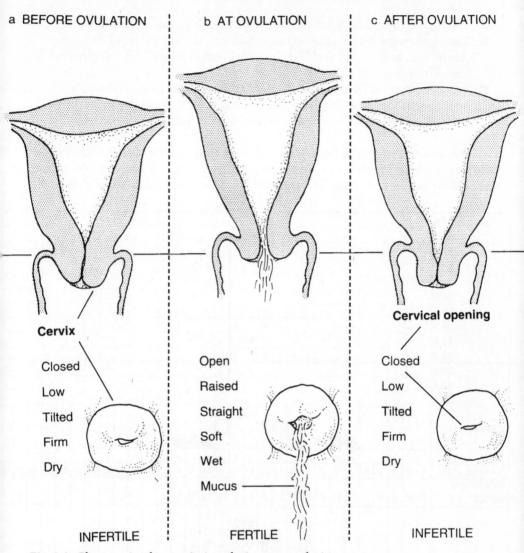

Fig 6.1 Changes in the cervix in relation to ovulation

SELF-EXAMINATION OF THE CERVIX

A woman can detect changes in the cervix by feeling gently with the finger-tip. A delicate touch is all that is required to distinguish the subtle day-to-day changes.

The cervix should be examined at the same time each day, for example while washing in the morning, after emptying the bladder. The same position should be used, either standing with one leg raised (for example, on the side of the bath), or squatting. If the position is varied then the cervix will appear to be at a different level.

- The hands should be washed and dried (the fingernails should be short).
- The right index finger is gently inserted into the vagina until the cervix can be touched. It will feel like a smooth indented ball. The vaginal walls feel soft, moist and ridged in comparison.
- If the cervix is difficult to reach, the uterus may be pushed down by pressing on the abdomen with the left hand, just above the pubic bone. With experience this examination should only take a few seconds.

Some women find it easier to use two fingers, the index and middle fingers, to examine the very subtle changes in the cervix. Other women find that their partner is more in tune with these changes and so is able to be

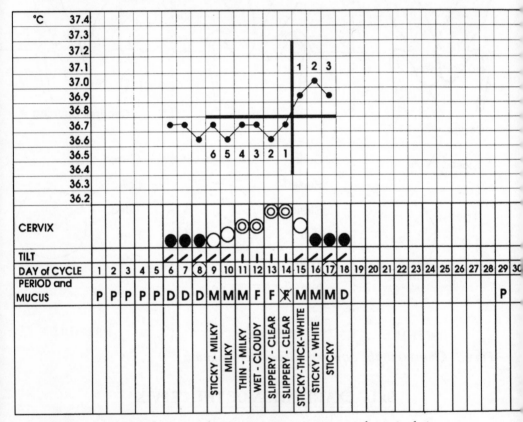

Fig 6.2 *Correlation between the temperature, mucus and cervical signs on a 28 day cycle. Onset of the fertile phase on day 9 is indicated by:*
i. *First observation of mucus*
ii. *First sign of change in cervix – softening*
To avoid pregnancy, the last intercourse was on day 8 and then not resumed until the post-ovulatory infertile phase was confirmed on day 17:
i. *Following the third high temperature past peak day*
ii. *After the cervix has reverted to its infertile state – low, firm, closed and tilted.*

actively involved and share the responsibility. It is important that cervical observations are made in the same way, by the same person. It generally takes two or three cycles for cervical changes to be interpreted accurately.

DETECTION OF MUCUS AT THE CERVIX
While checking the cervix, some cervical mucus may come away on the examining finger. This should be recorded on the chart separately.

Women who have difficulty distinguishing mucus changes externally or have a very short mucus build-up may find it useful to take mucus directly from the cervix in this way. This avoids the delay in transit time from cervix to vulva and gives an earlier warning of approaching fertility.

An interval of a day or two may occur before thick, sticky mucus noted at the cervix is visible externally. The more liquid, fertile mucus appears at the vulva within hours. Some women find that mucus becomes trapped in the ridged vaginal walls, and it appears as a long thread on the finger.

RECORDING CERVICAL CHANGES ON THE CHART

■ **The infertile cervix** is represented by a solid black circle drawn towards the lower end of the space to show that it is low, firm and closed. A slanted line below shows the tilt.
■ **The fertile cervix** is represented by an open circle to show softness, an inner ring shows the cervix to be open. A straight line below shows the cervix straight in position. The raised level of the fertile cervix is represented by the appropriate symbol being placed higher in the space.

Cervical signs may be helpful as a double check with mucus symptoms, especially at times when the temperature cannot be considered a reliable guide such as during illness. In such circumstances intercourse should not be resumed until the fourth evening after peak day which usually corresponds with the third evening of an infertile cervix.

The cycle in Fig 6.2 was recorded by an experienced user who has limited her observations to the necessary part of the cycle – from the end of the period (unless a woman has very short cycles) until post-ovulatory infertility is established. There is no benefit in continuing to record cervical signs or mucus symptoms during the post-ovulatory infertile phase, as this is both unnecessary and potentially confusing.

7. Minor Indicators of Fertility

PHYSICAL AND EMOTIONAL CHANGES DURING THE MENSTRUAL CYCLE

Hormonal fluctuations around the time of ovulation and pre-menstrually cause both physical and emotional changes. Signs may vary from one cycle to another, and different women will experience different symptoms, but each woman can learn to record these signals on her chart, increasing her awareness of fertility.

ABDOMINAL CRAMPS – OVULATION PAIN (ALSO CALLED MITTELSCHMERZ PAIN)

Many women will experience a sharp pain, or dull ache on one side of the lower abdomen lasting from a few minutes up to a few hours or longer. The cause of the pain is disputed. It may be due to muscular cramps in the uterus or the fallopian tubes or to the pressure of the distended follicle on the surface of the ovary. The timing of the pain can be a reliable indicator for some women, although others will find it very varied when correlated with temperature and mucus symptoms.

BREAST SYMPTOMS

Breast symptoms are very commonly experienced by women as an effect of either high oestrogen levels or high progesterone levels. The timing and the symptoms experienced will vary dependent on the hormone responsible.
- A characteristic tenderness or tingling sensation may be experienced around ovulation due to the high levels of oestrogen.
- When breast symptoms are experienced later in the cycle under the influence of progesterone, they are usually felt as a fullness and heaviness of the breast. These symptoms normally last until the onset of the next period.

SPOTTING OR LIGHT BLEEDING

A very small number of women may experience a few spots of blood or blood-tinged fertile mucus close to peak day. This is caused by the effect on the endometrium of a sharp fall in oestrogen levels around the time of ovulation. Spotting will occur while the temperature is still in the low phase (pre-ovulatory) or as the temperature shift is occurring. It indicates peak fertility and should not be confused with true menstruation which occurs at the end of the high temperature level. Spotting associated with ovulation is rare and any woman who has inter-menstrual bleeding should seek medical advice.

EFFECTS ON LIBIDO (SEXUAL DESIRE)

All women have a low level of male hormones (androgens) including testosterone in the blood. Around the time of ovulation there is an increase in these hormones, the function being to suppress the activity of the ovarian follicles. In some women the hormonal effect may increase the libido – nature's way of encouraging sexual activity at the time most likely to achieve pregnancy. Although this phenomenon is probably related to increased androgen and oestrogen activity, it is not a universal experience. Some research has shown that more women experience increased sexual desire in the pre-menstrual phase.

Changes in human libido are obviously also dependent largely on psychological and social factors. Couples using a natural method to avoid pregnancy may meet problems if a woman's sexual desire is increased at her fertile time and reduced pre-menstrually. It is important that couples are able to talk this through to avoid risk-taking behaviour, and find other ways of expressing love acceptable to them both.

THE LYMPH NODE SIGN

Some women may be aware of enlargement and tenderness of a small gland or node in the groin, occurring for a day or two around ovulation, at the peak of fertility. The gland is said to enlarge on the same side as the ovary that is ovulating. Vulval swelling may also be more marked on the side where the gland is felt. This sign which was first reported by Professor Erik Odeblad in Sweden in 1991 has not been used extensively, but for some women the appearance and disappearance of a pea-sized tender lump in the groin may be another minor indicator of fertility.

PRE-MENSTRUAL SYNDROME (PMS)

LORNA: Depression. The very word makes people feel low. Lorna suffered from severe bouts of depression, hard on her husband, bad for her children, Jean and Tim, and debilitating for herself. Sometimes she felt she was going mad.

Keeping charts really helped Lorna. She charted her temperature and mucus signs, and she also recorded her emotions, good days and days when she felt depressed. There on the chart, as clear as daylight, she could see that her bad days were related to her cycle. Depression started a week before her period, sometimes earlier but always ceased within 48 hours of the beginning of the period. She knew it was physical, and not 'all in the mind'. Lorna went back to her doctor, who recommended hormone treatment, which solved the problem for her and also for her family.

Pre-menstrual syndrome is the term used for a collection of symptoms which occur one to two weeks before a menstrual period. The symptoms disappear at the onset of menstruation. Pre-menstrual syndrome should not

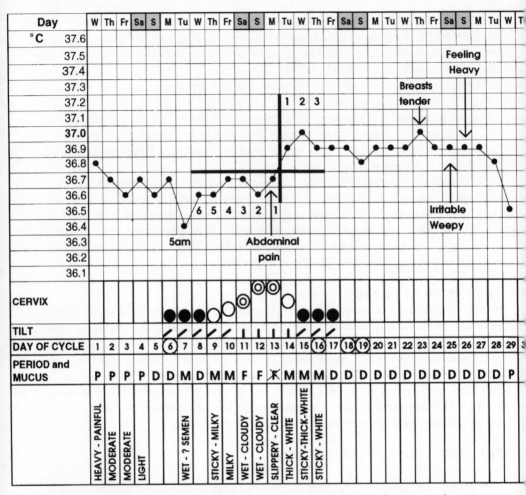

Fig 7.1 Inclusion of minor indicators. Note the abdominal pain on day 13 which coincides with peak day for this woman. Pre-menstrually she has noted breast tenderness, a heavy sensation and irritability.

be confused with dysmenorrhoea (painful periods), the symptoms of which appear the day before or at the onset of menstruation and disappear at its end.

Symptoms of pre-menstrual syndrome (often known as pre-menstrual tension or PMT) include irritability, nervous tension, mood swings, crying, depression, headache, loss of energy, breast tenderness, abdominal bloating weight gain and carbohydrate craving. The severity of the symptoms may vary from a nuisance value in mild cases, to causing serious disruption of family and social life in severely affected women.

If a woman is disturbed by cyclic symptoms, she should consult her doctor. Pre-menstrual syndrome may be associated with low levels of

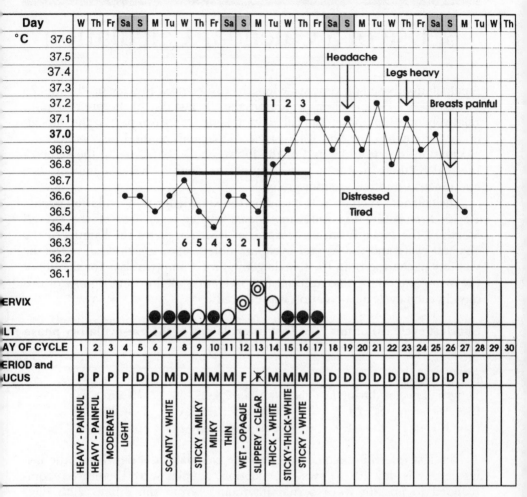

Fig 7.2 Marked pre-menstrual changes. This chart shows quite severe physical and emotional changes pre-menstrually affecting almost half of the cycle. Note the swinging temperature post-ovulatory – an indication of disturbance in the progesterone levels.

progesterone in the post-ovulatory phase. Progesterone therapy may be most effective for these women. Supplements of vitamin B6 or Evening Primrose oil have also proved beneficial for some women. Some doctors are now looking at dietary habits and stressing the advantage of regular meals, eating natural foods and restricting highly refined foods, sugar and stimulants such as tea, coffee and alcohol.

There are numerous theories about the cause of PMS, including hormonal, neurological, psychological, and social. As no one hypothesis can explain the variety of symptoms, likewise the appropriate treatment is also varied – from drugs and hormones, to dietary therapy and lifestyle and stress management.

8. Use of a Calendar Calculation

A calculation based on past cycle lengths can be used to back up the mucus symptom as a double check in identifying the last day of the pre-ovulatory relatively infertile phase. The calculation is derived from part of the old calendar or rhythm method. The original calendar method also includes a calculation to define the end of the fertile phase, but if using the sympto-thermal method, this is unnecessary as the double check of temperature and mucus symptom are more reliable.

The calendar method was based on the knowledge that ovulation occurs 12–16 days before the following menstruation regardless of the overall length of the cycle. From a record of at least six cycles the lengths of the shortest cycle and the longest cycle are noted. Allowing three days for the viability of the sperm in the female genital tract and two days for the life of the ovum and taking into account that ovulation might occur on any of five days in each cycle a calculation was evolved:

Shortest cycle (S) minus 20 = Last infertile day of the pre-ovulatory phase
Longest cycle (L) minus 10 = Last fertile day

For example:
Length of cycles during last six months = 28, 29, 28, 27, 30, 28
(S = 27)   S – 20   =   Last infertile day   27 – 20 = 7
(L = 30)   L – 10   =   Last fertile day   30 – 10 = 20

The last infertile day according to the calculation is day 7 and the last fertile day is day 20. To avoid conception, couples were therefore recommended to abstain from sexual intercourse from the 8th to 20th days inclusive. The calendar or rhythm method may give an unnecessarily long period of abstinence.

It is now known that the ovum can be fertilised only within a few hours of ovulation and the viability of the sperm in the genital tract is variable and may be longer than three days. Although the calendar method is not sufficiently reliable to be recommended for use as a single indicator, the information gained by recording the length of cycles and their variability is useful.

DETECTING THE EARLY INFERTILE PHASE BY A CALCULATION
The shortest cycle minus 20 calculation is most valuable for couples requiring a high degree of effectiveness, but wishing to have intercourse in the pre-ovulatory relatively infertile phase. During the learning phase many women have difficulty distinguishing the very early cervical mucus changes. The use of this calculation acts as an additional safeguard to warn of the onset of the fertile phase.

> **SHORTEST CYCLE MINUS 20 CALCULATION**
> Estimate the shortest cycle length over the previous year.
> For example, cycle lengths are 32, 29, 31, 30, 30, 29, 31, 29, 30, 31, 30, 29:
> Shortest cycle (S) is 29. Subtract 20 to give the last infertile day
> **S minus 20 = last infertile day**
> 29 – 20 = 9   Last infertile day is day 9

For many women the S minus 20 calculation will determine the end of the pre-ovulatory infertile phase a day or two before the warning given by first mucus symptom. However, if mucus is noted before the day designated by the calculation, this would indicate the onset of the fertile phase.

The S minus 20 calculation should be continuously reassessed to monitor the shortest cycle over the previous year by recording the current and the shortest cycle length at the top of each chart.

THE DOERING RULE

The Doering rule gives a slightly more accurate estimation of the onset of the fertile phase. It is based on calculations made from the day of the temperature shift, which generally follows within 24 hours of ovulation.

> **DOERING RULE**
> Identify the earliest temperature shift from the previous six cycles (12 if available).
> For example, temperature shifts on days 15, 16, 16, 17, 15, and 16 respectively:
> Earliest temperature shift is day 15
> Subtract seven days from this to give the first fertile day
> **Earliest shift day minus 7 = first fertile day**
> 15 – 7 = 8   First fertile day is day 8

The Doering rule can be used as an effective double check to identify the onset of the fertile phase as soon as a woman has recorded sufficient cycles. It has the advantage over the simpler calendar calculation in that it allows for variability in the luteal phase and is therefore more precise. It generally corresponds more closely with the onset of the mucus symptom. The fertile phase is indicated by the Doering rule or the earliest mucus symptom, whichever comes first.

The 'stop bar'

A 'stop bar' or solid vertical line can be drawn on the chart to designate either the end of the pre-ovulatory infertile phase calculated by the S minus 20 rule, or the beginning of the fertile phase calculated by the Doering rule. In Fig 8.1 (overleaf) the shortest known cycle is 28 days, therefore the stop bar is drawn after day 8 which is the last infertile day by the S minus 20 calculation.

CHART INTERPRETATION

The completed sympto-thermal chart can be interpreted using the following step-by-step guide.

Make your observations in the same order:

1. Check:
- Age of woman
- Number of chart
- Length of shortest cycle

2. Was the last temperature chart biphasic ?

3. Is this chart from a woman in special circumstances ?

4. Interpret the temperature chart:
- Length of cycle
- Day of shift
- Apply the rule of '3 over 6'
- Identify the first day of the post-ovulatory infertile phase

5. Interpret the mucus pattern:
- Identify the first appearance of mucus
- Interpret mucus pattern according to description
- Identify 'peak mucus day'
- Identify the pre-ovulatory and post-ovulatory infertile phases
- Double check mucus with temperature

6. Interpret changes in the cervix (optional):
- Low, firm, closed, tilted cervix is infertile
- High, soft, open, straight cervix is fertile

7. Apply the calculations if there is a record of at least six cycles:
- Shortest cycle minus 20 to identify the last infertile day
- Earliest shift day minus 7 to identify the first fertile day

8. Observe the timing of minor indicators

9. Check other factors which may affect the charts:
- Disturbances
- Stress factors
- Illness
- Medication

10. Apply the guidelines appropriately:
- For planning pregnancy
- For avoiding pregnancy

Colour code:
Coloured highlight pens can be used to aid chart interpretation, emphasising the phases of the cycle, for example:
- Red for the period
- Yellow for the fertile phase
- Green for the infertile phases

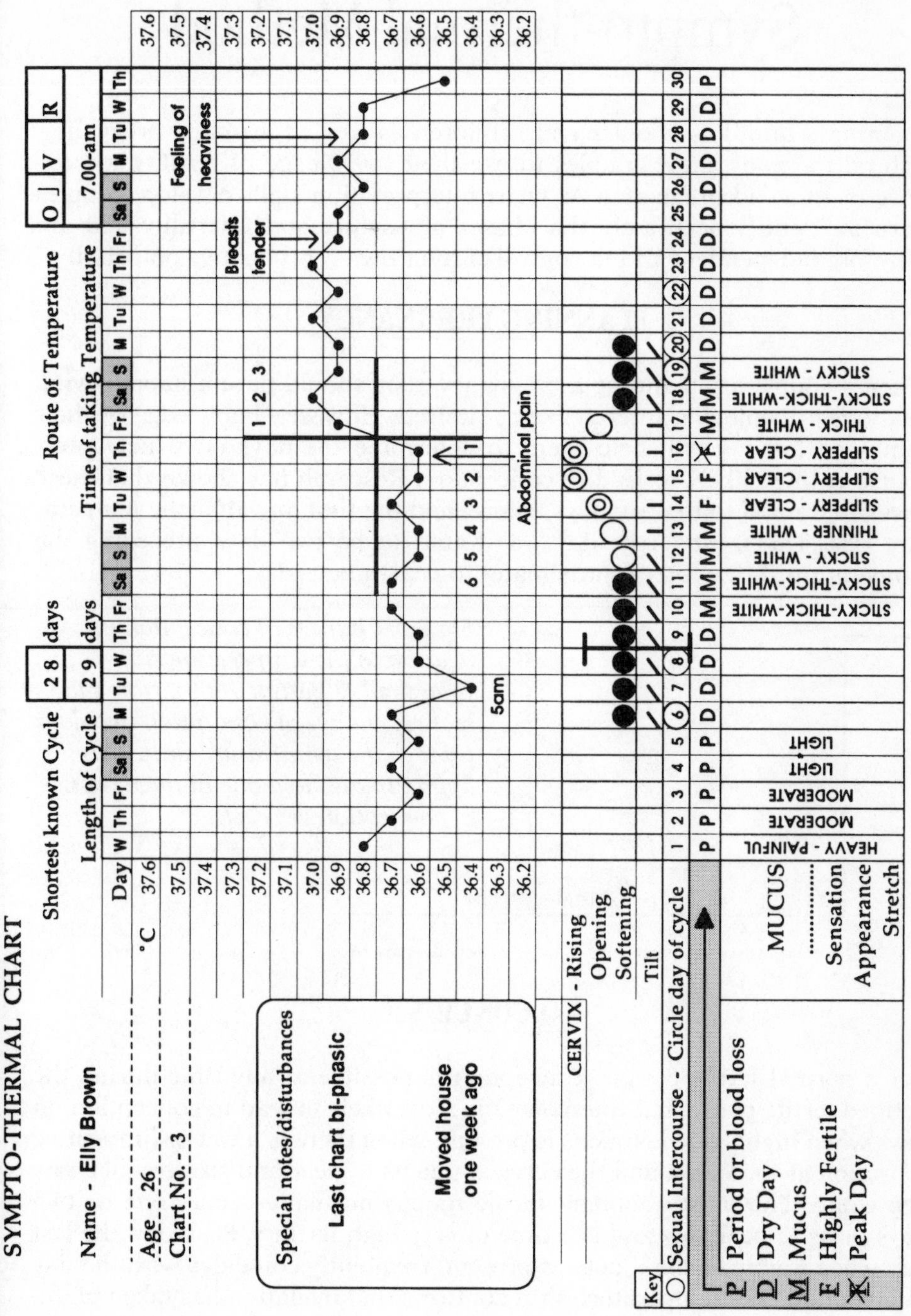

Fig 8.1 *Completed sympto-thermal chart showing correlation between all indicators of fertility*

9. Planning a Family by the Sympto-thermal Method

Planning a family is about having children as well as avoiding pregnancy. Natural methods allow couples to use their knowledge of fertility to conceive or to avoid pregnancy. As chart interpretation skills develop, couples learn to identify accurately the phases of fertility and infertility and are therefore independent and in control of their own reproductive potential.

PLANNING PREGNANCY

When a couple are planning a pregnancy, they should have a happy loving relationship, enjoying intercourse as desired. However, knowledge of their combined fertility will help them to determine the days on which intercourse is most likely to lead to conception. Research has shown that these days are limited to the five days before, and the first day after the temperature rise. The most fertile day was found to be two days preceding the temperature shift which approximates to peak mucus day.

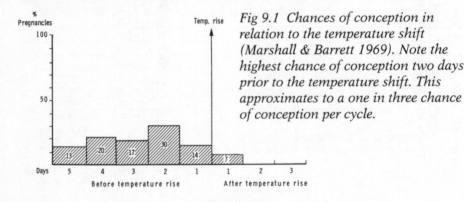

Fig 9.1 Chances of conception in relation to the temperature shift (Marshall & Barrett 1969). Note the highest chance of conception two days prior to the temperature shift. This approximates to a one in three chance of conception per cycle.

TO CONCEIVE

For a normal fertile couple, conception is possible at any time during the defined fertile phase, but intercourse is most likely to lead to conception on days when highly fertile mucus is present, when there is a wet or lubricative sensation at the vulva, and the cervical mucus is clear and stretchy like raw egg white. The most abundant fertile mucus normally occurs one or two days prior to peak day and is a time of very high fertility. Peak day, the last day when highly fertile mucus is present, frequently coincides with the day of ovulation. The temperature shift confirms that ovulation has taken place. At the time of maximum fertility, the cervix is high, short, straight, soft, open and flowing with fertile mucus.

GUIDELINES TO CONCEIVE

Aim to have sexual intercourse during the fertile phase :
- ■ When highly fertile mucus is recognised.
- ■ As close to peak mucus day as possible.

A couple who have not achieved pregnancy after six months (following regular intercourse at the fertile time of the cycle) should see their general practitioner, who may advise further investigations.

VALUE OF THE TEMPERATURE IN CONFIRMING PREGNANCY

In a cycle where conception occurs, a woman may record a second increase in temperature, to an even higher level, several days after the ovulation shift. This is due to an increase in progesterone production following implantation. A raised temperature lasting more than 20 days almost certainly indicates pregnancy. A pregnancy test can be done to confirm this.

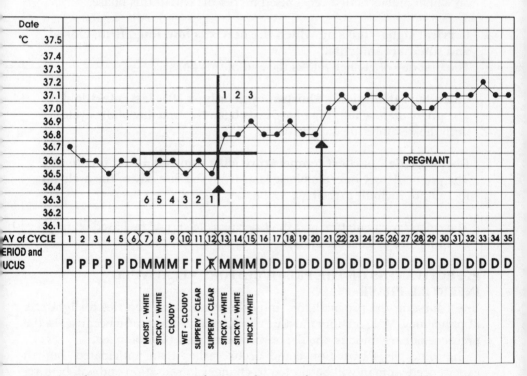

Fig 9.2 Achieving pregnancy. This couple were planning a pregnancy. Intercourse on day 12 in the presence of fertile mucus was followed by a temperature shift, shown by the first arrow. The second arrow shows the further shift in temperature. The sustained high temperature for over 20 days confirms pregnancy.

AVOIDING PREGNANCY

Couples using a natural method to avoid pregnancy, whether to space or to limit their family, must learn to identify accurately the limits of fertility and to apply the appropriate guidelines. Integrating abstinence into a sexual relationship requires the commitment and co-operation of both partners.

GUIDELINES TO AVOID PREGNANCY
Pre-ovulatory relatively infertile phase

The pre-ovulatory relatively infertile phase can be identified by the mucus symptom, cervical signs, a calendar calculation or the Doering rule. It is advisable to have a double check and to consider the onset of the fertile phase as given by the earliest indicator.

Mucus symptom – following the period, dry days are infertile.
It is wise to restrict intercourse to alternate evenings, because the presence of seminal fluid in the vagina may mask cervical mucus. The day on which mucus is first recognised marks the end of this phase.

Cervical signs – days on which the cervix is low, long, firm, closed and tilted are infertile.
The first day of change marks the end of this phase.

Calendar calculation – Shortest cycle minus 20 = last infertile day.
The pre-ovulatory infertile phase lasts from the first day of the cycle until the last infertile day inclusive.

Doering rule – earliest temperature shift minus 7 = first fertile day.
The pre-ovulatory infertile phase lasts from the first day of the cycle up to, but not including, the first fertile day.

The calendar calculation and the Doering rule should be based on information from at least six cycles.

EFFECTIVENESS OF THE PRE-OVULATORY RELATIVELY INFERTILE PHASE

Intercourse in the pre-ovulatory infertile phase always carries a slight risk of pregnancy. Male fertility must be considered in this phase because, in the presence of early mucus, the life of the sperm may be prolonged.

In some cases ovulation could occur earlier than anticipated, but an experienced woman will be alerted to changes in sensation and will be forewarned of an early ovulation. In a very small number of women, with short cycles of around 21–24 days, or with prolonged menstrual bleeding, mucus may appear immediately after the period or even before its end. In this case intercourse during a period could lead to conception – there will be no pre-ovulatory relatively infertile phase.

GUIDELINES TO AVOID PREGNANCY
Post-ovulatory infertile phase

The post-ovulatory infertile phase can be confirmed by the temperature, mucus or cervical signs.

Temperature – after the third high temperature has been recorded provided:
■ All three high temperatures are undisturbed.
■ At least one is a minimum of 0.2°C above the coverline.
■ There is a minimum of six low temperatures.

Mucus symptom – on the fourth evening after peak day.

Cervical signs – on the third day after the cervix has returned to its infertile state.

USING THE SYMPTO-THERMAL METHOD
The post-ovulatory infertile phase starts:
after the third high temperature
has been recorded provided that
all three high temperatures are past peak mucus day.

EFFECTIVENESS OF THE POST-OVULATORY INFERTILE PHASE
It should be emphasised that the post-ovulatory infertile phase is the safest time for intercourse for a couple wishing to avoid pregnancy. When ovulation has been confirmed there is no risk of further fertility in the current cycle.

Where there are very serious contra-indications to pregnancy, couples may choose to wait an extra day. Intercourse should be avoided until the evening of the fourth day of higher temperature readings before assuming infertility. If the mucus pattern is not recognised, infertility should not be assumed until the evening of the fifth day of higher temperatures to avoid any misinterpretation of the temperature shift. These 'life or death rules' according to Dr Joseph Roetzer are as reliable as male or female sterilisation.

SUMMARY OF GUIDELINES TO AVOID PREGNANCY

The fertile phase starts at the
first mucus symptom or the first day by calculation, whichever is earlier,
and lasts until the
third high temperature past peak day.

KATE AND QUENTIN: *Kate attended an interest talk on fertility aware-ness hoping to learn where she had gone wrong. She and Quentin had not intended to start a family, not yet. She had read the Billings book and from that had taught herself to observe the mucus signs. She had obeyed the rules, so why was she pregnant?*

Kate was interested to learn about the sympto-thermal method and at the end of the talk she arranged an appointment for herself and Quentin to see one of the NFP teachers. She took her charts with her and it was clear that observation of mucus only two days before 'peak', gave insufficient warning of approaching ovulation.

Since the birth of their baby, Kate and Quentin have had no prob-lems in using a natural method of family planning. Using the Doering rule to identify the end of the pre-ovulatory relatively infertile phase, the mucus signs and the temperature chart to identify the beginning of the post-ovulatory phase, they have found the method reliable. Their second child was planned and conception occurred as expected.

WHY VARIOUS NFP ORGANISATIONS USE DIFFERENT RULES

During the last 25 years, programmes for teaching natural family planning have been implemented in more than 90 countries throughout the world. Various organisations have been engaged in this work. Each organisation has produced its own charts and teaching material and has developed its own guidelines for identifying the fertile and infertile phases of the cycle. These guidelines reflect the emphasis laid on efficiency and acceptability for peoples of different cultures. The number of days of abstinence will vary according to the flexibility of the rules. Some organisations will sacrifice a degree of efficiency to allow a method which is culturally and practically acceptable. In India, the modified mucus method is used extensively as it is felt necessary to reduce the time of abstinence in order to obtain a wider number of users. Abstinence is limited to the days of slippery stretchy mucus and two days and nights after peak mucus day.

The Billings method allows intercourse on the evenings of alternate dry days in the pre-ovulatory infertile phase and unrestricted intercourse in the post-ovulatory infertile phase from the fourth day after peak mucus symp-tom. Intercourse must be avoided during menstruation.

The Hilgers ovulation method, or Creighton model, has similar rules to Billings but uses a special mucus scoring system. Women wishing to learn the Creighton model must be instructed by specially trained teachers.

HOW THE LENGTH OF ABSTINENCE VARIES ACCORDING TO THE NATURAL METHOD USED

Where mucus-only methods are used to prevent pregnancy, the length of abstinence in the pre-ovulatory phase depends on the length of the period, the number of dry days and the type of mucus observed.

The length of abstinence required by couples using the sympto-thermal

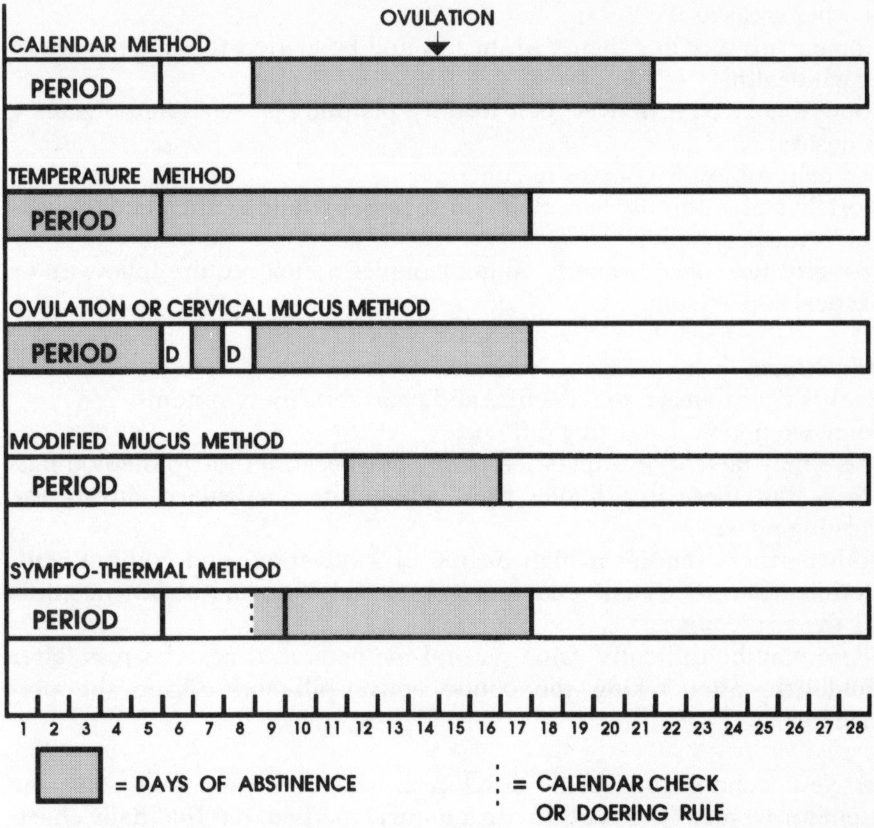

Fig 9.3 *The length of abstinence required by different natural family planning methods. This shows a hypothetical 28 day cycle for a woman who has cycles ranging from 28–31 days.*

method will vary according to the strictness of the guidelines used. Some couples will require the highest degree of efficiency and will be prepared to abstain for longer to achieve this. Other couples may be in a position to relax the guidelines allowing more time for intercourse. The motivation for avoiding pregnancy will be stronger at some stages during the reproductive lifespan than at others and couples can adopt guidelines to suit personal circumstances.

ADVANTAGES AND DISADVANTAGES OF NATURAL METHODS OF FAMILY PLANNING
Advantages
■ No interference with the woman's normal physiology.
■ No known physical side effects.
■ Both partners share the responsibility for planning their family. The education necessary for fertility awareness may lead to better communication and may contribute to a more co-operative relationship

in other areas as well.

■ Women can monitor their own health and be alerted to any changes in sexual health.

■ Couples have control over their fertility, planning or avoiding pregnancy as desired.

■ Can help subfertile couples to conceive.

■ Morally and culturally acceptable in societies where artificial contraception is unacceptable.

■ Cost-effective: once properly taught, couples do not require follow up or medical supervision.

Disadvantages

■ It takes time to learn to recognise and chart fertility symptoms.

■ Some women find charting difficult.

■ There may be fear of unplanned pregnancy because though method failure is low, there is a higher user failure rate particularly during the learning phase.

■ Both partners require a high degree of motivation, and commitment. Modifications to sexual behaviour are needed to ensure abstinence during the fertile phase.

■ There may be difficulty using natural methods at times of stress, after childbirth, after taking the contraceptive pill and during the premenopause.

Note: New technology is being developed, which will hopefully solve the problem for women who wish to use a natural method, but find daily charting tedious or difficult.

10. Effectiveness

COMPARISON OF NATURAL FAMILY PLANNING WITH CONTRACEPTIVE METHODS

When considering the effectiveness of any form of family planning, the distinction must be made between:
- the theoretical or method effectiveness (the biological effectiveness).
- the practical or use effectiveness (the behavioural effectiveness).

Since the 1930s the accepted measure of contraceptive effectiveness has been the pregnancy rate per 100 women-years of use, according to the Pearl Index. This shows how many women would get pregnant if 100 women used a given method of family planning for one year.

Family planning method	Theoretical or method failure	Practical or user failure
Male sterilisation	0.15	0.1
Female sterilisation	0.4	0.5
Hormone implant	0.09	<1–2
Injectable	0.3	<1–2
Combined pill	0.1	<1–3+
Progestogen-only pills	0.5	1–4+
IUS	0.4	<1
IUD	0.6	<1–2
Condom	3	2–15
Sympto-thermal method	1–3	2–15
Female condom	5	2–15
Diaphragm/cap with spermicide	6	4–18
Withdrawal	4	19
Spermicides	6	21

Table 10.1 Comparative efficiency of different methods of family planning taken from a wide range of studies.
Source: FPA, Trussel et al 1990

The theoretical or method effectiveness is the maximum effectiveness of the method when used without error or omission, that is when used according to the instructions. In theory the failure rate for the sympto-thermal method, for example, is around two per cent.

The practical or use effectiveness takes into consideration all users of the method, that is those who follow the method without error and also those who are less committed and less consistent in their use. It denotes the effectiveness under real life conditions – for example the sympto-thermal method has a user failure rate of 2–15 per cent.

A couple's motivation has a crucial influence on the use effectiveness of a number of methods of family planning. The first year's use always carries the highest risk of unplanned pregnancy due to the time taken for a couple to learn to use the method efficiently. Barrier methods require some skill and a high degree of motivation and pills are more frequently forgotten during the first year of use.

EFFECTIVENESS OF NATURAL FAMILY PLANNING

Study		Natural family planning methods	Description of study	Participants	Method failure	Overall user failure
Ball	1976	Ovulation		122	2.9	15.5
WHO Auckland, Dublin, Balangore, Manila, San Miguel	1980	Ovulation	Multicentre Trial	869	2.8	19.6
			TEACHERS			
Perez	1981	Ovulation	Inexperienced			16.4
Chile	1982		Experienced			2.6
Wade USA	1979	Ovulation Sympto-thermal	Comparative Study			24.8 9.4
Johnston, Roberts & Spencer USA	1978	Ovulation Sympto-thermal	Comparative Study	268 586		27.6 15.9
Parenteau-Carreau, Lanctot, & Rice Canada	1976	Sympto-thermal	TOTAL Spacers Limiters	168 67 101	0.7	6.0 14.9 1.1
Rice, Lanctot, & Garcia-Devesa Canada	1979	Sympto-thermal		1,022		7.5
John Marshall UK	1982	Sympto-thermal	Experienced Users	108	0.3	3.9
Barbato Italy	1986	Sympto-thermal	New Users	460 Couples	2.0	3.6
Clubb, Pyper & Knight UK	1988	Sympto-thermal	New Users	72	1.3	2.7
Freundl & Frank Germany (ongoing)	1993	Sympto-thermal	New Users	506	0.5	2.3

Table 10.2 Natural family planning efficiency studies

A high degree of motivation is essential if a couple are to use natural methods of family planning successfully. They should both be in accord about their goals of family spacing or limiting. It is interesting to note that the family-spacers, those who plan more children but at a later date, are less effective in preventing pregnancy. They are prepared to take risks; whereas family-limiters, those who have completed their family, are more conscientious and determined, and more successful in preventing pregnancy. This is illustrated in Table 10.2 by the 1976 Canadian sympto-thermal study which showed a failure rate of almost 15 per cent for the family-spacers and around one per cent for those limiting their families.

The 1978 American study comparing the sympto-thermal with the ovulation method shows the sympto-thermal method to be almost twice as effective, because there is less chance of making an error when there is a double check available.

It is vital that couples are taught by NFP teachers who are appropriately trained and updated and offer high quality instruction. In the early 1990s, the Chilean study followed a group of teachers after their initial training course, monitoring their efficiency during their first year's teaching experience, and again a year later. They showed a dramatic improvement in the teacher-related failure as they gained experience.

The effectiveness of any form of family planning depends on the method being well taught, well understood and well applied, but this is of particular importance for natural family planning. With experience, the sympto-thermal method is a highly effective method. This is illustrated by the more recent sympto-thermal studies. The degree of efficiency afforded by the sympto-thermal method depends on the guidelines used.

PRE-OVULATORY RELATIVELY INFERTILE PHASE

Pre-ovulatory infertile days can be efficient if the pre-ovulatory calculation S minus 20 (or preferably the Doering Rule) is checked against the observation of the first mucus symptom.

A 1984 study, by Dr Anna Flynn, of eight experienced users of the sympto-thermal method concluded that the most reliable indicator to detect the beginning of the fertile period was the calendar calculation, S minus 20. Mucus was not always present sufficiently early to warn of approaching fertility. One pregnancy resulted from intercourse on a dry day which was calculated by ultrasound scan and hormone assays to be five days before ovulation. If the S minus 20 rule had been applied it was reasonably assumed that the pregnancy might not have occurred, as sexual intercourse would have been discontinued two days previously.

The couple who accept the slight possibility of pregnancy may use the pre-ovulatory infertile days. Since unplanned pregnancies usually arise from intercourse in this phase and during the first two years of use of the method, the inexperienced couple should be advised not to use these days before they are confident in determining the onset of the fertile phase.

POST-OVULATORY INFERTILE PHASE
The post-ovulatory infertile days ensure the highest degree of efficiency. Beginners in the method should use only the post-ovulatory infertile days for intercourse. It is helpful if the instructor can identify the late infertile phase with the couple for the first two or three cycles, or until they feel sufficiently confident to determine this alone. Adding a day or two to allow for misinterpretation of the peak mucus day will increase the rate of success in the learning phase.

In the 1982 Marshall study, which included women with normal fertile cycles and women in special circumstances, where the overall failure rate was 3.9 per cent, there were no pregnancies after the third high temperature was recorded. More recent European sympto-thermal studies have confirmed the very high degree of efficiency of the post-ovulatory phase.

EFFECTIVENESS OF TEACHING NFP IN GENERAL PRACTICE
A community-based project was carried out in a NHS health centre in Oxford, to assess the efficiency and cost-effectiveness of teaching the sympto-thermal method. A practice nurse used group teaching and audiovisual aids. During the project, 72 women wishing to avoid pregnancy charted 903 cycles with an overall failure rate of 2.7 per cent on the Pearl Index. In this study there were 26 couples with fertility problems wishing to conceive; 19 were successful. The cost per patient based on four hours' teaching was £27.90 in 1988. The updated cost at 1995 is £39.95 for the first year's cost. Subsequent cost of charts, replacement thermometers or further teaching due to changing fertility status is minimal.

The cost of teaching NFP compares favourably with other methods. Those couples who continue with the method, using it efficiently to prevent unplanned pregnancy, achieve large savings for family planning providers. This is particularly significant in the developing world.

Contraceptive pill	£111.43
Diaphragm	£112.20
IUD	£205.10
Spermicide	£118.95
Injectable	£123.71
Implant	£367.12
Condom	£64.29
Sympto-thermal method (4 hours' teaching)	£39.95

Table 10.3 Comparative cost with other methods of contraception per annum
Adapted from: 'The economics of family planning services', Mcguire and Hughes/FPA. A report prepared for the Contraceptive Alliance, 1995

The numbers of couples using natural methods in Europe is increasing for ecological, ethical or medical reasons, but many of these couples gain information from friends or books and have no formal instruction. There is still opposition from some members of the medical profession and only highly motivated couples are strong enough to challenge this and to use a natural method.

The effectiveness of natural family planning as shown by the recent European studies is now recognised and couples who wish to use a natural method need have no anxiety about an unplanned pregnancy, provided they are taught by an experienced teacher and are sufficiently motivated to keep strictly to the guidelines.

11. After Childbirth and During Breast-feeding

BREAST-FEEDING

Women who choose to breast-feed their babies will be able to take advantage of the weeks or months of infertility, when intercourse will not lead to pregnancy. This is known as the Lactational Amenorrhoea Method (LAM), which is now being recommended internationally. However, research in general practice among women who have had children has shown that the majority of those who start to breast-feed give up after a few weeks because of problems which need never occur. The women did not want to be pressurised, but wanted to decide for themselves whether to breast-feed their babies or not. It is quite possible for mothers who choose to bottle feed to use a natural method of family planning. Normal fertile cycles will return within a few weeks and the guidelines they have already learned will apply.

The following information about breast-feeding can help women to make informed choices :

■ Breast-feeding is the natural way to space a family. Amongst the peoples of developing countries, there is far more effective family planning from breast-feeding than from all other methods of artificial contraception. The World Health Organisation has been alarmed by the rapid increase in population in countries where artificial (bottle) feeding has been introduced.

■ Mother's milk is the best food for her baby; not only does it contain all the essential, easily digested proteins, lactose and the cream to give the necessary nourishment, but it has other unique properties that no other milk can supply. At the beginning of a feed the milk is thin and clear. The extra water content satisfies the baby's thirst. At the end of a feed the milk has become rich, with five times more cream. This helps to regulate the baby's appetite and gives complete satisfaction.

■ Breast milk contains the antibodies needed to protect the baby against infection and also protects the child from some allergies.

■ There are advantages to the mother in breast-feeding. Breast-feeding is good for her health and for her figure. Stimulation of the breasts by the nursing baby will cause reflex contractions of the uterus preventing pro-longed blood loss and discharge, and promoting a rapid return to normal physiology. During pregnancy the average weight gain is about 12 kg/26 lb. One third of this is the energy reserve for producing breast milk. A breast-feeding mother will lose weight and so regain her figure more quickly, provided she eats sensibly.

■ Breast-feeding helps to develop the bonds of affection between mother and baby, and within a few days the breast-fed baby will recognise his own mother and turn towards her.

BREAST-FEEDING PROBLEMS

Breast-feeding should be a happy experience for the mother, but too often problems arise – sore or cracked nipples, tender breasts or a fretful unsatisfied baby – and breast-feeding is abandoned in favour of the bottle. These problems are unnecessary and should never occur if the mother receives help when she starts to breast-feed her baby.

Firstly it is important to realise that the nipple does not fill with milk like the teat on a bottle, so the baby must not suck the nipple (which causes pain and soreness), but must open his mouth wide to take in the whole of the coloured area of the areola and so draw milk from the breast through the nipple. If the baby is properly positioned at the breast, there should be no problems. Breast-feeding will be a satisfying experience for mother and child, and the parents will be able to rely on this natural time of infertility to resume sexual intercourse without anxiety about another pregnancy.

ZOE AND SCOTT: Visiting the UK from America, Zoe was expecting her first baby within the month. Though sorry to be so far from home, she was looking forward to the birth. She was confident all would go well. Her pregnancy had been easy, and she had prepared well for a 'natural birth'. In the event, labour was prolonged and she had a forceps delivery. The baby was beautiful and a good weight, but poor Zoe suffered a number of complications. To add to her misery, she found breast-feeding extremely painful. After her return home, a Sister from the hospital with expertise in helping breast-feeding mothers visited her, and helped her to position the baby on the breast correctly. From that time, she was without pain, and happy breast-feeding her son.

RESEARCH

Research studies have been carried out among the Eskimos and among the rural Indians of North America where no other form of contraception was being used, and where there was no taboo on sexual intercourse during lactation. The time taken for 50 per cent of the women to conceive again was six months in those artificially feeding, but an average of 18–24 months among the breast-feeders.

In 1981 Professor Howie and others carried out research on mothers to compare the return of fertility among bottle-feeders and breast-feeders. The mothers who were bottle feeding had all resumed ovulation and menstruation by 15 weeks, averaging a return of fertility between nine and 13 weeks postpartum (after the birth). But among the breast-feeding mothers, he found that there was no ovulation during total breast-feeding and that ovulation and menstruation were delayed for a variable length of time during weaning. Howie found that ovulation occurred early among those women who suckled infrequently, introduced supplements rapidly and stopped night feeds. By contrast, those in whom ovulation was delayed, maintained night feeds, introduced supplements slowly and cut down the frequency and length of suckling time gradually. In the first group, ovulation occurred rapidly after weaning was started, around 16 weeks, but in the second group, the return of fertility in some women was delayed for up to 15 months or longer. Howie found that ovulation did not occur among breast-feeding mothers who gave at least five feeds, totalling 65 minutes a day.

PHYSIOLOGY

Following childbirth, all women produce large amounts of the hormone prolactin, which stimulates the production of breast milk. Prolactin also effects the hormones which control the fertility cycle. Prolactin acts on the pituitary, interfering with the action of follicle stimulating hormone (FSH) and luteinising hormone (LH) and thereby reducing the production of oestrogen. The low level of oestrogen during breast-feeding suppresses the maturation and ripening of the follicles and thus prevents ovulation. Within hours of delivery, there is an increase in the sensitivity of the nerve endings in the nipple so that each act of suckling stimulates the secretion of pro-lactin. The level falls again after 3–4 hours, but if the baby suckles frequently, including short spells of comfort suckling, the high level of pro-lactin is sustained, thus preventing ovulation.

LACTATIONAL AMENORRHOEA METHOD (LAM) OF CHILD SPACING

LAM is based on WHO sponsored research. At a conference held in Bellagio in 1988, a consensus document was produced which concluded that a woman is 98 per cent protected from pregnancy when:
- She is fully or almost fully breast-feeding.
- The baby is less than six months old.
- Menstruation has not returned.

Fully breast-feeding means that the baby is fed by his mother on breast milk alone without the addition of other milk, fruit juices or solid foods. Water may be given. Almost fully breast-feeding means that the mother is giving no more than one or teaspoonfuls of other foods. In either case the baby will be fed on demand and will suckle for nourishment and comfort instead of having a dummy or pacifier. This frequent suckling is important to maintain infertility during lactation. It is interesting that the Kung hunter-gatherers of the Kalahari desert have an unusual pattern of suckling: not 10 or 20 minutes from each breast every four hours, but for a few seconds or a couple of minutes four times an hour.

As a result of ongoing research in many countries, it is realised that even

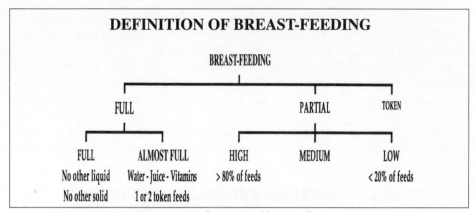

Fig 11.1 *Definition of breast-feeding*

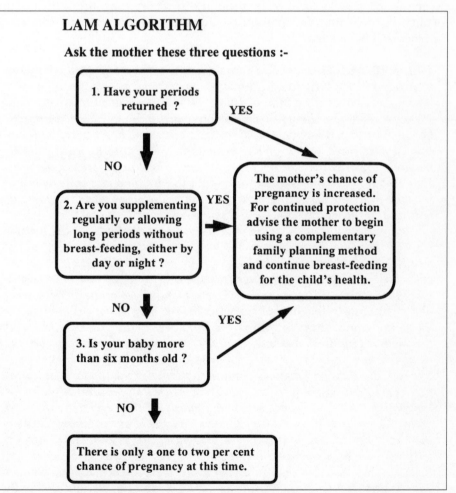

Fig 11.2 *Use of Lactational Amenorrhoea method for child spacing*

when weaning starts, the breast-feeding mother may still be protected against pregnancy. To maximise this effect, it is recommended that the breast-feeds should be given before any supplements.

Promoters of LAM recognise that mucus patches may be difficult to interpret and the method requires long periods of abstinence, which may be found unnecessary in retrospect. LAM does not require mucus observation, but simply that the above criteria are met. Any change, for example over six months after the birth, return of menstruation or the introduction of weaning, increases the chances of pregnancy and necessitates sympto-thermal charting.

FERTILITY AWARENESS DURING BREAST-FEEDING

If a woman was already aware of her fertile pattern before she became pregnant she should have little difficulty in recognising the return of her fertility, but learning the method during breast-feeding means that much patience will be needed.

JILL AND DONALD: Jill and Donald had wanted a big family, but they were happy with their four children under six and wanted to call a halt. Spacing, as far as it had happened at all, was a result of breast-feeding. However, Thomas, the youngest, had weighed 4.54 kg/10lb at birth. Jill had developed varicose veins and her blood pressure had been raised during the last three weeks of her pregnancy. She came to learn natural methods towards the end of breast-feeding. The teacher was concerned. Here was a client who should on no account become pregnant, wanting to learn from the beginning, at a time when the signs and symptoms of fertility and infertility would be difficult to recognise.

Jill was adamant she wanted to use natural methods, so the teacher insisted that Donald must attend as well, even if it meant bringing all the family. The first session was a long one. Donald and Jill were glad to discuss their problems, their feelings for each other and for their family, and to explain their attitudes to marriage and family planning. They were willing to abstain for the necessary time while they learnt the method. At the next session, fitted in during the same week, Jill and Donald learnt the basis of natural methods and the rudiments of charting. Mucus recognition was a problem which continued long after Thomas was weaned. But Jill's periods had become regular, and the biphasic temperature chart allowed them to use just the post-ovulatory infertile phase for intercourse. Jill also learnt self-examination of the cervix. In the next cycle, she not only found it easy to recognise the changes taking place on the chart, but for the first time she recognised the crystal-clear stretchy, fertile mucus as it appeared like a thread when she withdrew her finger. So seven months from their first visit to the NFP teacher, Jill and Donald were independent and confident in using a natural method of family planning.

RECOGNISING THE BASIC INFERTILE PATTERN

After childbirth, there will be several weeks of blood-stained discharge, known as the lochia. This diminishes and gives way to a recognisable state of infertile mucus discharge, or dryness. The recognition of her infertility is as important to the breast-feeding mother as awareness of fertility.

MUCUS SIGNS – THE BASIC INFERTILE PATTERN
- Dry days are infertile.
- Moist days. A constant pattern of mucus may be experienced giving a moist sensation. Provided that this mucus is unchanging day after day for over two weeks, this can be regarded as the infertile mucus pattern (BIP of mucus). The mucus may be thin, white and milky, or there may be a slight stickiness only or a yellowish discharge. The essential thing to establish is its unchanging characteristics. Any dry days found during a pattern of unchanging mucus are infertile.

TEMPERATURE
The temperature will be swinging, that is, the day-to-day variation will be greater. It may be at a different level, often lower than in a normal fertile cycle. This is characteristic of the infertility associated with breast-feeding. As there may be many months of infertility during breast-feeding, some individuals may prefer to rely on mucus alone, or a combination of mucus and cervical changes. The advantages of keeping a temperature record during the breast-feeding period should be explained. The swinging temperature is a sign of infertility, which many women find reassuring, and as her fertility returns the temperature pattern will level, and ovulation will be recognised by the temperature shift.

CERVIX
The cervix will return to its normal state about 12 weeks following the birth. After this time a woman may start recording changes in the cervix. She should be aware that after the birth of a baby, particularly the first baby, the cervix will not feel exactly as it did in the pre-pregnant state. The os will not close as completely, even in its infertile state, and may admit the fingertip. Significant changes related to fertility will however be apparent.

RECOGNISING SIGNS OF APPROACHING FERTILITY

Once the basic infertile pattern has been established any change in the mucus symptom or in the cervix could signify approaching fertility.

MUCUS
- If the infertile pattern was of dry days, any change from the sensation of dryness or any visible mucus would signify possible return of fertility.

- If the basic infertile pattern was of moist days, the pattern will change. There may be a change in sensation, to produce a wet or slippery feeling, or changes in quantity, colour or consistency of the mucus. Fertile-type patches of mucus may be noticed, without ovulation taking place. This may be regarded as an attempt at ovulation, as oestrogen levels fluctuate. As fertility approaches the mucus is likely to appear more frequently.

TEMPERATURE

The temperature will level. A Canadian study by Dr Suzanne Parenteau-Carreau (1983) found that in a significant number of women the temperature levelled for one or more weeks before the shift. This could therefore supply a further valuable warning sign of impending ovulation in breast-feeding women.

CERVIX

Changes in the cervix may give the earliest information of approaching fertility. The cervix rises higher in the vagina, becomes straighter and softer, and opens up.

RECORDING ON THE BREAST-FEEDING CHART

The breast-feeding chart (see pages 92–3) should be used to record as much information as possible about mother and baby. Each chart covers eight weeks.

BABY

1. The number of feeds per day and the approximate suckling time should be calculated. Extra fluids or solids should be recorded.
2. The longest interval between feeds over 24 hours should be noted.
3. A record should be kept of baby's appetite, alterations in suckling vigour, general health, including teething, immunisation etc.

MOTHER

1. Basal body temperature should be recorded.
2. Mucus signs (sensation, observation and finger-testing) must be recorded. Observations should be made throughout the day and recorded in the evening.
- Dry days are marked with a **D**.
- Moist days forming the basic infertile pattern of mucus (BIP) are marked with an **m**.
- Days of sticky white mucus ie change from dryness or change from BIP of mucus are marked with an **M**.
- Fertile-type mucus days are marked with an **F**.
- Any bleeding is marked with a **P**.
3. The cervix may be examined each morning and changes recorded.
4. General health and any stress should be recorded, and taking alcohol or

drugs should also be noted. (All medication should be prescribed by a doctor who is aware that the mother is breast-feeding.)

5. If milk is expressed to give to the baby at a later stage (for example if the mother has to leave him/her for a while), a note must be made on the chart.

6. Any change in circumstances, such as a holiday, should be recorded.

USE OF COLOUR TO AID CHART INTERPRETATION

- The basic infertile pattern can be highlighted in green.
- Any change from the infertile pattern (days when fertility signs are present) can be highlighted in yellow.
- Yellow can be extended to include days when intercourse could result in pregnancy – for example for three days following return to BIP.
- Days of bleeding can be highlighted in red.
  The use of colour in this way clearly shows the pattern of infertility and potential fertility on the breast-feeding chart.

FACTORS WHICH MAY PRECIPITATE THE RETURN TO FERTILITY

- When breast-feeding becomes less frequent.
- The introduction of mixed feeding. This includes extra drinks of fruit juice or artificial milk and the introduction of small amounts of solid food. Ovulation and conception are more common after a sharp decrease in suckling time and frequency. Abrupt weaning can therefore result in a rapid return of fertility.
- When the baby first sleeps through the night (prolactin levels fall sharply).
- Anxiety, stress or illness – either in mother or baby. Unlike menstrual cycles where stress tends to delay ovulation, during breast-feeding the effect of stress is to allow ovulation to occur earlier than it might otherwise. Prolactin is inhibited, the oestrogen levels rise and fertile cycles return much sooner.

SHORTENED POST-OVULATORY PHASE IN FIRST CYCLE AFTER CHILDBIRTH

The interval between ovulation and the first menstruation following childbirth is often shorter than usual. It may be as short as 8–10 days. Cycles in which the post-ovulatory or luteal phase is less than nine days are infertile, as there is insufficient time for implantation.

Spotting or light bleeding may occur due to a rise in oestrogens around the time of ovulation, so a woman should not automatically assume that the first bleeding is menstruation.

In 60 per cent of women, the first sign of fertility will be blood loss, which has not been preceded by ovulation (anovulatory episode).

GUIDELINES TO AVOID PREGNANCY DURING BREAST-FEEDING

Use the coverline technique to identify the temperature shift

Prior to first ovulation
Mucus symptom
Identify the basic infertile pattern:
■ Continuous dryness or
■ Unchanging mucus pattern (established over at least two weeks).
If the BIP is dryness – any mucus is potentially fertile.
If the BIP is mucus – any change signifies fertility.
This pattern can be assessed towards the end of the time covered by the LAM criteria.

Cervical signs
■ Days on which the cervix is low, firm, closed and tilted are infertile.
■ Any change from the infertile state signifies fertility.

Temperature
■ Swinging temperature with great day to day variations indicates infertility.
■ Levelling temperature indicates impending fertility.

It is wise to restrict intercourse to alternate evenings during the pre-ovulatory phase.
At the first sign of returning fertility, whether shown by the cervix or the mucus, intercourse should be avoided while the fertile signs last, and for **three days** after the basic infertile pattern has returned.

Any day of bleeding is potentially fertile, as there is a possibility of the bleeding being associated with ovulation. Intercourse should be avoided on these days and for the following **three days**.

After the first ovulation post-natally
In the first cycle after childbirth, intercourse may be resumed after the **fourth** high temperature past peak day. The post-ovulatory infertile phase lasts until the start of the next period. The luteal phase may be shortened.

Subsequent cycles
Post-ovulatory infertile phase
In subsequent cycles, intercourse may be resumed after the **third** high temperature past peak day has been recorded. A couple can enjoy unrestricted intercourse day or night until the onset of the next period.

Pre-ovulatory relatively infertile phase
Guidelines for normal fertility should be resumed. The basic infertile pattern of mucus only applies prior to the first ovulation following childbirth. In subsequent cycles, only dry days can be considered relatively infertile.
The S minus 20 or the Doering rule must be re-calculated following resumption of normal fertile cycles. Evidence from cycles prior to childbirth should not be relied on.

AVOIDING PREGNANCY DURING BREAST-FEEDING

After the lochia has dried up, there are often episodes of vaginal blood loss as breast-feeding becomes established. This is quite common for up to six weeks. A couple can resume intercourse as soon as the woman feels comfortable and ready, which may take up to two to three weeks. There is no need to wait until after the post-natal check. There are no restrictions on intercourse while LAM guidelines apply (see pages 84–5).

If LAM indicates increased risk of conception, guidelines for intercourse in the pre-ovulatory relatively infertile phase should be followed.

WEANING AND ITS EFFECTS ON THE RETURN OF FERTILITY

If the baby is totally breast-fed, weaning usually occurs in the UK between four and six months. If weaning takes place gradually, this gives both mother and baby time to adjust. There may be several patches of fertile-type mucus before ovulation occurs. The pattern may seem confusing for a while. This is a time for great patience and co-operation between partners.

Fertility may return at the beginning, during, or at the end of weaning. The time taken for fertility to return, whether ovulation precedes the first menstrual period, or whether bleeding occurs with no preceding temperature shift, varies from woman to woman.

Breast-feeding should be a pleasurable, relaxed experience for both mother and baby. As a woman records her breast-feeding experience and state of infertility, she will gain confidence in knowing how her body is reacting to influences from her baby, and the environment. Throughout this time, intercourse should be enjoyed without any anxiety about conception.

Fig 11.3 (overleaf) Breast-feeding chart from 26–33 weeks after childbirth. The woman has established a BIP of dryness. The swinging temperature and the low, firm, closed, tilted cervix confirm her infertility. Supplementary feeds are introduced during the 27th week. Sticky mucus patches during the basic infertile pattern of dryness are potentially fertile and are followed by the count of three days before infertility is assured. There is no evidence of ovulation.

Fig 11.4 (overleaf) Breast-feeding chart continues from weeks 34–41. As supplementary feeds are increased, the number of breast-feeds are reduced. Note the levelling of the temperature followed by the shift in the 40th week. The arrows show the earliest sign of fertility as indicated by the cervix or the mucus. Mucus patches are observed more frequently, then copious amounts of slippery, clear, stretchy mucus are observed leading up to ovulation. The post-ovulatory infertile phase starts after the fourth consecutive high temperature past peak day. The coverline has been extended back to cover the low phase temperatures that have levelled. The post-ovulatory phase is slightly shortened.

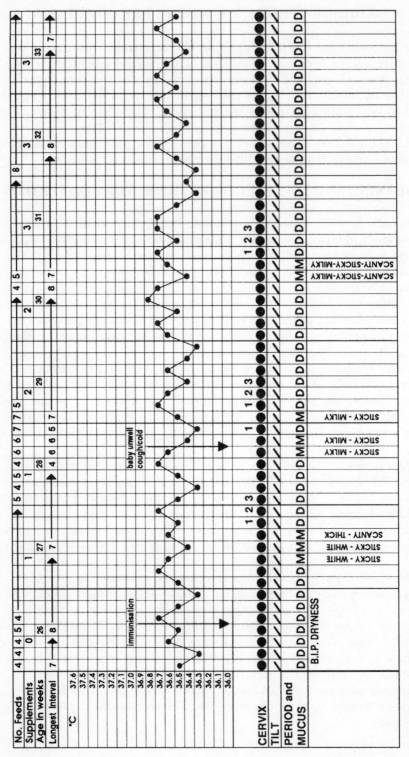

Fig 11.3 Basic infertile pattern during breast-feeding

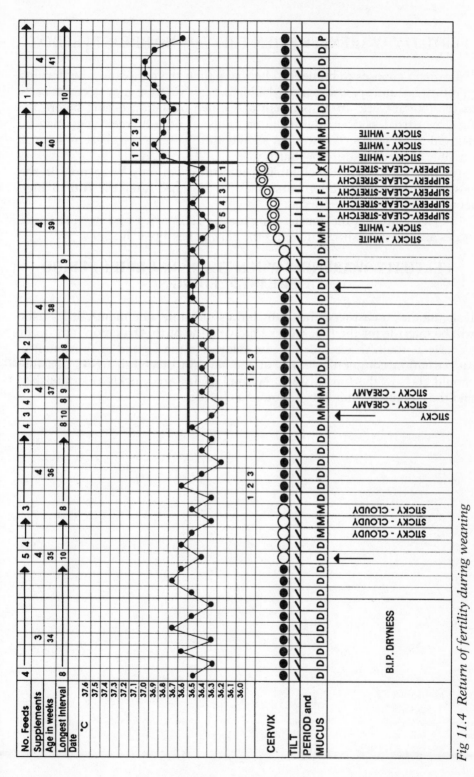

Fig 11.4 Return of fertility during weaning

FERTILITY AWARENESS WHEN THERE IS NO BREAST-FEEDING

If a woman chooses to bottle feed her baby then she may expect her fertility to return around six weeks after the birth, but ovulation may occur as early as the fourth week. In 50 per cent of women ovulation occurs before the first menstrual period. Menstruation is usual at 6–8 weeks but may be delayed to 10 weeks. The woman should start to keep her chart as soon as possible around the third or fourth week.

In the first cycle after childbirth, infertility can only be assured in the post-ovulatory phase. Intercourse may be resumed after the **fourth** high temperature has been recorded.

Subsequently, as the mucus symptom is recognised and normal fertile cycles are re-established guidelines for normal fertility will apply.

FERTILITY AWARENESS WHEN THERE IS A BRIEF PERIOD OF BREAST-FEEDING

If the mother breast-feeds her baby for a short time, one month or less, she will be infertile for the four weeks following the birth. Ovulation may occur as early as the fifth week or may be delayed to the second or third month. Menstruation commonly occurs at the seventh or eighth week. Charting should start in the fourth week. Normal cycles are quickly re-established and the guidelines should be followed as before.

12. Post-pill Users

The pill, the most widely used method of contraception, has many advantages as a highly efficient method of birth control. However, many women are concerned about potential side effects which are pill-related. Women who have not found pills acceptable for a number of reasons will often say how well they feel after stopping their pills and find many hidden benefits.

LINDA AND BOB: Linda and Bob had two children, Jean aged four and Bobbie aged two. Bobbie was born with a severe congenital heart condition and needed constant care. Linda was taking the pill because she knew she could not cope with another baby. She was very overweight and had raised blood pressure. The doctor advised her to use another method of family planning. She was reluctant to use barriers and had not been happy with an IUD. So she came to learn a natural method. Her teacher explained that, as she was coming off the pill, she would have to use strict guidelines, necessitating lengthy periods of abstinence, until her normal physiology returned. She was quite happy about this as she said that they only had intercourse about twice a month, and only then for her husband as she had lost all interest in sex. Four months later, Linda had lost two stone, her libido had increased dramatically and she looked radiant again. Linda was happy that she had found a method of family planning that worked for her.

PHYSIOLOGICAL CHANGES

The contraceptive pill causes a physiological disturbance in a woman's body. During the months after taking the pill, physiology is affected to a greater or lesser extent, possibly due to retained synthetic hormones.

THE EFFECTS OF COMBINED PILLS
Combined pills containing oestrogen and progestogen act mainly by preventing ovulation. After stopping the combined pill, there is often a rapid return to normal physiology with ovulation occurring within two weeks. In some women ovulation can be delayed for a few weeks or for several months. If hormone levels are fluctuating, there may be a number of attempts at ovulation. Oestrogen levels may rise sufficiently to cause mucus changes, but may not reach the necessary level to trigger ovulation. The progestogen component of the pill stimulates the production of thick mucus, which is impenetrable to sperm. The mucus pattern may be affected for a while after stopping combined pills, though this effect is often more marked with progestogen-only pills.

Cyclic Changes

There are many variations to be expected after stopping the pill. Some women will recognise normal fertile symptoms very quickly, others will find disturbances lasting for several months and still others will notice an apparent return to normal fertility with disruption later. The following cyclic changes are commonly seen post-pill, in some cases for up to a year or longer. The possible combinations are endless.

Variations in cycle length and in the pre- and post-ovulatory phases

- Long, normal length and short cycles.
- Variations in shift day.
- Short post-ovulatory phases, around 8–10 days.
- Anovulatory cycles.

Effects on mucus pattern

- Persistent dry days.
- Unchanging mucus pattern.
- Continuous scant sticky mucus.
- Continuous watery or milky pattern.
- Erratic mucus patches of varying types of mucus.
- Heavy mucus flow.
- Mucus symptoms not in relation to temperature shift.

Other pill-related problems which may affect mucus observation

- **Cervical erosion or ectropian**

If there is an excessive mucus discharge after two cycles, a woman should see her doctor. There is an increased incidence of cervical erosion caused by the effects of the pill and also following childbirth.

- **Candidiasis or thrush**

Some research indicates a slightly higher incidence of thrush in pill users. This is generally seen as a curdy, white, irritating discharge, which can be treated quickly and effectively, usually by pessaries prescribed by the doctor.

Effects on temperature

- False high temperatures not related to ovulation.
- Temperature and mucus signs not correlating.

While taking the pill it is not possible to learn fertility awareness, but women who record temperatures during pill use will notice it is on one level – monophasic – and usually at a slightly higher level than the normal, post-ovulatory phase, due to the progestogen in the pill. This raised temperature normally falls after pills are stopped, but it may take a time to settle, giving false readings.

Changes in vaginal bleeding

Some women will complain of heavy bleeding after coming off the pill. The withdrawal bleed while taking the combined pill is generally a lighter flow, so a woman may have become accustomed to the lighter periods associated with pill use. She may also notice a change in the colour of her blood loss from a dark red/brown colour to the brighter red loss of her true menstrual period.

Bleeding can only be recognised as a true period if preceded by a temperature shift approximately 14 days before. If bleeding occurs without a temperature shift in the preceding cycle, it may be due to hormonal fluctuations associated with ovulation and must therefore be regarded as a sign of fertility. In such circumstances, recordings should be continued on the same chart, as this is still the pre-ovulatory phase. A new chart is started at the beginning of a true period.

RECOGNISING A TRUE PERIOD
■ A true period is preceded by a temperature shift around 14 days previously.
■ Any bleeding not defined as a true period is potentially fertile.

THE EFFECTS OF PROGESTOGEN-ONLY PILLS
The main action of the progestogen-only pill in preventing pregnancy is to cause changes in the cervix, keeping it hard, tightly closed and plugged with thick sticky mucus which prevents sperm penetration. Progestogen-only pills prevent ovulation in over 60 per cent of cycles. Many cyclic changes associated with combined pills may be observed by women discontinuing the use of hormonal products containing progestogen-only.

After stopping this type of pill, there is frequently considerable disturbance to the mucus pattern. This effect may also be noted with other progestogen-containing injections, devices, or implants.

Changes in the mucus pattern
The mucus pattern will vary from woman to woman but most frequently there is a heavy flow of mucus for many days of the first cycle, diminishing to a normal number of mucus days and a more recognisable pattern by about the third cycle. The mucus frequently shows a continual watery or milky pattern, producing a wet sensation throughout. Sometimes there may be scant, sticky, mucus – either as an unchanging pattern or occurring as patches of mucus.

Each individual's mucus pattern will be different. Cervical mucus may be excessive and not in relation to the temperature shift, making it difficult to interpret the peak symptom. Rarely it may take up to six months or even longer for the woman's normal fertile pattern to return after coming off the progestogen-only pill.

This failure highlights the problems that can arise during the months after coming off the pill. Women should be warned of the possibility of long cycles during which ovulation may be delayed for many weeks. Unplanned pregnancies commonly occur when a couple tire of waiting for signs of fertility or the temperature shift, and assume the cycle to be anovulatory. Couples who have learnt to use natural methods effectively during normal fertility should always seek further support when they notice any cyclic change. This is particularly important post-pill.

HELEN AND TONY: Helen and Tony had used natural methods when they were first married but then finding difficulty with abstinence in their new relationship, they decided to change to the pill. Unfortunately Helen started to suffer from recurrent migraines and she was advised to stop the pill. She and Tony disliked other contraceptives and so decided to try natural methods again but they ran into problems. Helen could no longer recognise her mucus. She seemed to have a continual watery or milky discharge and there were three cycles with no temperature shift. On the fourth chart there was still no shift and by the 25th day they decided (wishful thinking) that this was going to be another anovulatory cycle. They had intercourse that night. The temperature shift occurred two days later and Helen was pregnant.

RECORDING ON THE POST-PILL CHART

Commence charting as soon as possible after stopping the pill. The first day of the cycle is the first day of post-pill blood loss. The normal fertility chart can be used which covers 40 days but remember that post-pill cycles can be very long. If this occurs two charts can be cut and aligned to aid interpretation.

GUIDELINES TO AVOID PREGNANCY POST-PILL

Use the coverline technique to identify the temperature shift
First cycle
Even if the cycle appears normal, there is no discernible infertile phase, due to the effects of the pill.
INTERCOURSE MUST BE AVOIDED THROUGHOUT THE FIRST CYCLE

Second cycle
The post-ovulatory infertile phase can be used for intercourse, starting from the **fourth** day of the higher temperatures, provided they are **all** a minimum of 0.2°C above the coverline.
INTERCOURSE MUST BE AVOIDED IN THE PRE-OVULATORY PHASE

Third and subsequent cycles
The post-ovulatory infertile phase starts after the **third** high temperature has been recorded, provided they are all past peak mucus day. Intercourse should

---

be restricted to the post-ovulatory infertile phase, until there is a recognisable mucus pattern which coincides accurately with the temperature shift.

Pre-ovulatory relatively infertile phase

When normal fertility has returned, the pre-ovulatory relatively infertile phase may be used for intercourse using the guidelines for normal fertility.

■ Period or bleeding

Intercourse is permitted during a period, provided that it is a true period confirmed by a preceding temperature shift. There is always a relative risk of pregnancy owing to an early ovulation.

■ S minus 20 calculation

This should be re-calculated after normal fertile cycle have returned. It cannot be relied upon for at least one year after discontinuing the pill.

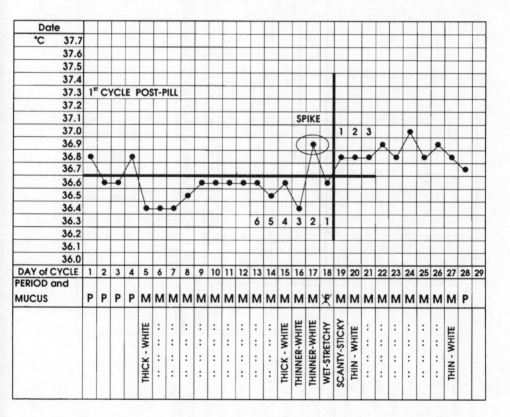

Fig 12.1 First cycle post-pill: apparently normal fertile cycle lasting 27 days. The biphasic chart is confirmed using the coverline technique. The luteal phase is slightly shortened. There is copious thick white mucus with only day 18 showing more fertile mucus characteristics. In spite of an apparently discernible temperature shift, the post-ovulatory phase cannot be considered infertile. There is no recognisable infertile phase during the first post-pill cycle.

Fig 12.2 Fourth cycle post-pill. This cycle demonstrates the importance of using the extended coverline to identify the temperature shift. There is a possible temperature shift on day 14 at the time it may have been expected, but although there are six low temperatures, the shift is minimal. The true temperature shift confirming ovulation occurs on day 23. The high temperatures are a minimum 0.2°C above the coverline which can be extended backwards over all the low phase temperatures, excluding the first four days of the cycle.

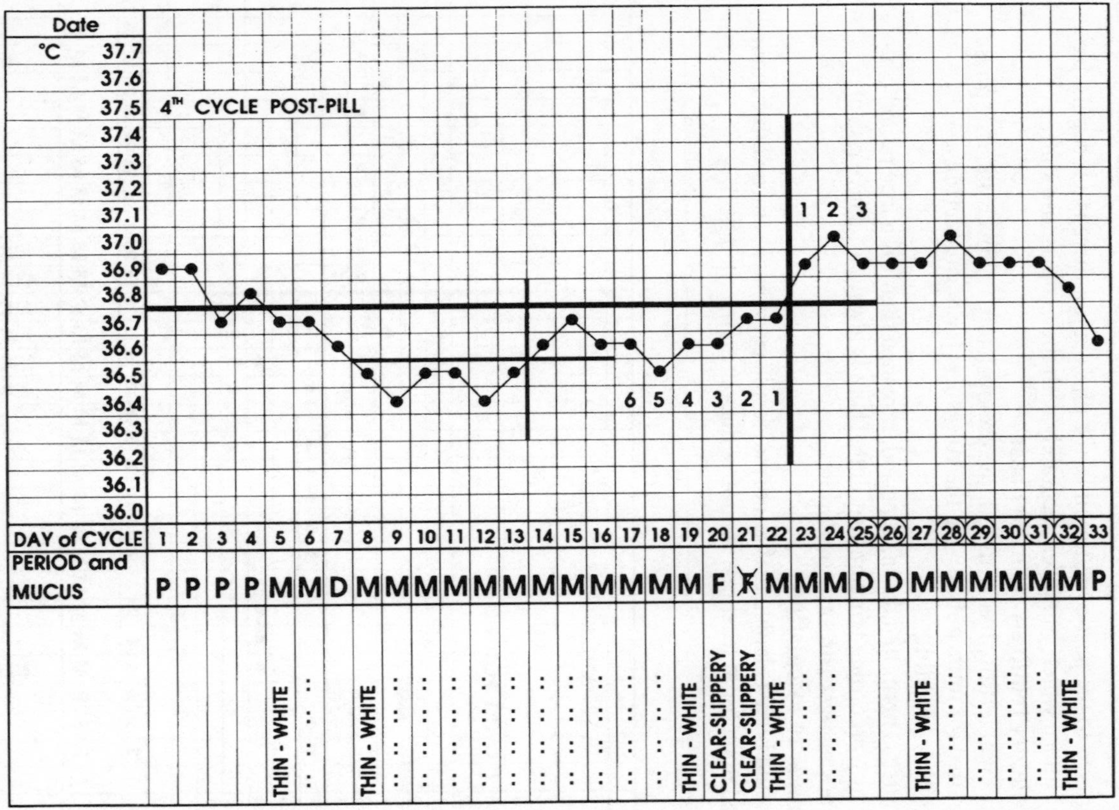

4TH CYCLE POST-PILL

DAY of CYCLE	1	2	3	4	5	6	7	8	9	10	11	12	13	14	15	16	17	18	19	20	21	22	23	24	25	26	27	28	29	30	31	32	33
PERIOD and MUCUS	P	P	P	M	M	D	M	M	M	M	M	M	M	M	M	M	M	M	F	✗	M	M	M	D	D	M	M	M	M	M	M	M	P

Mucus observations: THIN-WHITE, CLEAR-SLIPPERY, THIN-WHITE

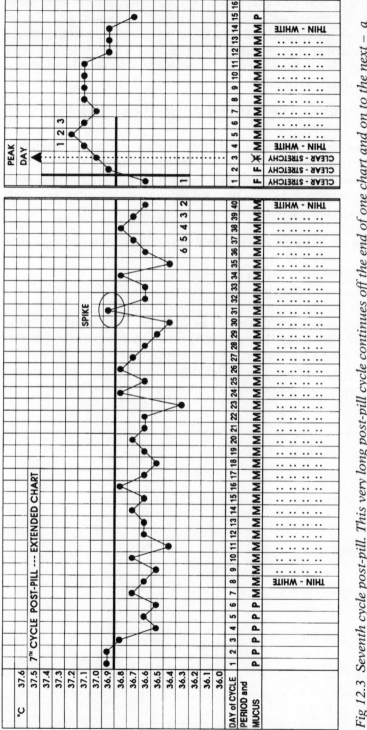

Fig 12.3 Seventh cycle post-pill. This very long post-pill cycle continues off the end of one chart and on to the next – a none too rare occurrence, particularly post-pill. The cervical mucus is a continuous thin white secretion showing more fertile characteristics from day 41, leading to peak on day 43. The temperature is quite erratic but, using the coverline technique, the shift can be seen on day 42. Correlating the temperature with the mucus symptom, as the peak day occurs after the shift, the post-ovulatory infertile phase does not start until day 46, that is after three high temperatures past peak day.

Some women will find cycles return to normal very quickly after stopping the pill but others will find tremendous variation and cyclic disturbance. The series of post-pill charts on pages 99–101 demonstrate some of the irregularities, the sequence and timing of which will vary from woman to woman. Cyclic irregularities do not appear to be related to the type of pill, or the duration of pill use.

PLANNING PREGNANCY AFTER COMING OFF THE PILL

In the past it has been recommended that women wishing to conceive should wait for at least three months after coming off the pill, to allow time for the resumption of normal physiology. Fertility clinics are now suggesting that the first three months can be used to conceive as there is a high chance of conception during this time.

To maximise the chances of conception, intercourse should coincide with:
■ Any days on which fertile mucus is present.
■ As close to peak day as possible.

Although for many women there will be little or no delay in returning fertility, the Oxford FPA study (Vessey, 1986) found that impairment of fertility was greater among women over 30, particularly among those women who had never had a child. Despite reduced fertility for a year or longer in some cases, he found no evidence suggesting that the pill causes long-term irreversible infertility.

13. The Pre-menopausal Years

Natural physiological changes occur throughout life. A child becomes an adolescent, the adolescent becomes an adult. Changes occur with pregnancy, childbirth and motherhood, but it is these last few years of a woman's fertile life that are often referred to as 'the change of life'. These years of the pre-menopause start for most women around the age of 45 and last until the end of reproductive life, when menstruation, the monthly periods, will cease. This is the true meaning of the word menopause and occurs between 50–55 years for the majority of women. The menopause, it should be stressed, only marks the end of a woman's fertility; her femininity is unaffected.

There is no reason why this 'change' should be more dramatic or more traumatic than those already experienced, but like other changes, it may bring its problems, physical, psychological or emotional.

In the UK one woman in eight is aged between 45–55 years old. The positive approach to maintain well-being and good health is very important. There is a clear relationship between a healthy body and an easier menopause. It is important to understand what is happening to your body at this time. Ignorance about what to expect will lead to unnecessary anxiety. Every women should have access to information and medical advice to make sure that these years, far from being unhappy, are a time of contentment and good health.

PSYCHOLOGICAL ASPECTS OF THE PRE-MENOPAUSE

The natural changes are not only physical but there may also be psychological and emotional stress on a woman. Family situations may cause problems. As her children grow up they will inevitably face adolescent crises in one form or another. They may be leaving home, or embarking on marriage themselves. Emotional stress may be aggravated at this time by the ill-health or death of elderly relatives.

A woman's husband may have his own problems adapting to changing circumstances. The prospect of retirement may be a daunting one. Although men do not go through a physical or hormonal change in the way that women do, the psychological effect of the 'male menopause' cannot be denied. Communication is an essential element at every stage in a relationship, but during the 'change' partners have a particular need of each other's love, understanding and mutual support.

If a woman has a positive outlook, she can plan future activities when there will be more time for her to develop her career or to spend on hobbies and interests. A woman who has worked in her own home may consider returning to some form of outside employment. A woman who is financially independent may have a more positive outlook on life, and the changes associated with the menopause will be minimised.

Circumstantial changes may be beyond a woman's control, but a knowledge and awareness of the body's changes can dispel fears at this time. Talking with friends who have been through, or are going through the menopause may be of help, others may find help from women's support groups.

PHASES OF THE PERI-MENOPAUSE
(time around the menopause)

PRE-MENOPAUSE
These are the years before menstruation ceases, when oestrogen and progesterone levels are diminishing. The lower levels of hormones are planned – women do not suffer from a deficiency disease at this time. Women over 40 may begin to notice some cyclic disturbance including menstrual irregularity and increasing numbers of anovular cycles. This may be the start of the transition towards the menopause.

MENOPAUSE
- Ovulation and menstruation cease.
- Production of progesterone ceases and oestrogen levels fall.

Since fertility is dependent on ovulation, not menstruation, a woman over 50 can assume permanent infertility after six consecutive anovulatory cycles. Even if she is still menstruating either regularly or irregularly, there will be no possibility of pregnancy. A woman under 50 should wait for 12 consecutive anovulatory cycles, before permanent infertility is assumed. For further confirmation, a doctor can check a woman's pituitary hormone levels. When FSH reaches a certain level, this shows that the ovary is not responsive and the woman will no longer be fertile.

POST-MENOPAUSE
There is no release or only a very minimal production of ovarian oestrogen. Other organs such as the adrenal glands and the body fat continue to produce oestrogen, thus feminine characteristics are maintained. The levels of FSH and LH are substantially elevated in the early post-menopausal years and these high levels often reduce in later years.

PHYSIOLOGY OF THE PERI-MENOPAUSE

All female babies are born with their complement of ova (eggs) for life. No more than 390 of these cells will mature and no other ova will be formed in later life. Ova deteriorate slightly with age, hence the increased risk of chromosomal disease, such as Down's Syndrome, in babies born to older mothers. As the ovaries cease to function in mid-life, this reduces the risk of substandard eggs being fertilised.

During a woman's most fertile years, in each cycle there are up to 30 follicles maturing in the ovary. Their combined efforts supply enough oestrogen to stimulate the process leading to ovulation.

During the pre-menopause, as a woman reaches the time when her reproductive function ceases, the ovaries produce fewer follicles. Less oestrogen is produced and attempts at ovulation will be, therefore, less successful.

As the production of oestrogen by the ovary decreases, the pituitary gland increases the production of FSH in an attempt to stimulate the ovaries. One of two things may happen:

- The follicles respond – the oestrogen levels rise, the endometrium is thickened, fertile mucus is produced and ovulation occurs. Ovulation may occur early resulting in a short cycle. The period may be heavy and prolonged.
- The follicles fail to respond – less oestrogen is produced, the follicle will not mature and rupture, ie no ovulation. The cycle will be long, the period short with minimal loss.

The pattern of cycles will vary from woman to woman, and also from year to year for the same woman. Finally the ovaries are no longer able to respond even to the increased stimulation. The hormone production will be too low to allow menstruation and ovulation. No oestrogen is produced by the ovaries after the menopause.

However, the production of oestrogen does not stop altogether after the last menstruation. The adrenal glands and body fat manufacture and store oestrogen. This is slowly released into the circulation. It may take a year or so for the adrenal glands to take over producing a baseline of oestrogen. In the meantime, the male hormone testosterone (of which small amounts are present) is unopposed by oestrogen and may contribute to feelings of irritability and aggression.

As the progesterone levels fall, the post-ovulatory phase is often shortened (8–10 days). Even if ovulation does occur, the corpus luteum is often inefficient and unable to sustain pregnancy. Eventually no more progesterone is produced.

SYMPTOMS COMMONLY FOUND PERI-MENOPAUSALLY

The following list of symptoms are associated with a decrease in oestrogen levels. Not all women will experience symptoms to an extent which causes problems, in fact 20 per cent of women go through the menopause without problems. If a woman is aware of the kind of symptoms to expect and understands their cause, she will see them in perspective and realise when medical advice is needed, and when symptoms are natural and should cause no anxiety.

The menopause may be welcomed by those women who have previously suffered from painful periods or pre-menstrual symptoms. If breast tenderness was a marked feature in cycles before, it may disappear altogether during the pre-menopause.

PRE-MENOPAUSAL SYMPTOMS
Menstrual irregularity
For some women, menstrual periods will stop suddenly and without trouble, but the majority of women will experience some irregularity, including 'missed periods' when very long cycles occur. There may be heavy prolonged menstrual flow with clots, due to over-stimulation of the endometrium.

Cystitis (infection or inflammation of the bladder)
This causes frequent, painful urination. It commonly occurs among the young – hence 'honeymoon cystitis'. It may occur pre-menopausally due to slight loss of elasticity in the urinary tract tissue. Self-help measures include drinking plenty of fluids, taking mild pain-killers and resting with a hot-water bottle to ease the pain. Medical advice should be sought if symptoms persist.

Vaginitis
This is a condition of dryness, soreness and irritation of the vagina and vulva which may make intercourse painful. Unhurried lovemaking, possibly with the use of a non-irritant water-soluble lubricating jelly, will help to overcome this. Lower oestrogen levels cause thinning of the vaginal lining, making inflammation and infection more common. Vaginitis responds well to medical treatment including hormone creams.

Hot flushes
These are brief events caused by sudden and transient dilation of the blood vessels, during which a feeling of heat suddenly rises up the body to the head, producing redness of the neck and face and generalised perspiration which quickly subsides.

Flushes may be occasional, or in extreme cases up to 30 flushes a day, then none for several weeks. They may happen day or night, in severe cases causing sleep disturbance. Flushes are frequently intensified by stress. Hot flushes are harmless and will pass. If they are slight they should be ignored. Lighter clothing, lighter bedclothes and a cooler atmosphere will help. They may cause a woman embarrassment but she should remember that other people will notice little or nothing.

Palpitations
These may be experienced as the heart fluttering, or a pounding sensation in the chest. There may be transient weakness. Palpitations may accompany hot flushes or occur alone. If they are disturbing, medical advice should be sought.

Weight increase
This is common during the pre-menopause years. It may be exaggerated by emotional factors leading to overeating and to lack of physical exercise. If a

woman becomes excessively overweight, other symptoms may be aggravated. Calorie requirements decrease with age but, although less food is needed, the diet must still contain all the essential nutrients to maintain a healthy body.

Tiredness, insomnia, headaches, backache, nervousness, depression, memory loss and generally feeling unwell

These may all have a contributing physical cause and should be checked by the general practitioner.

Note: The above symptoms are transient and usually disappear around the time that menstruation ceases.

POST-MENOPAUSAL SIGNS AND SYMPTOMS

Osteoporosis

This is a condition caused by a decrease in oestrogen levels, where the bones become more brittle due to lack of calcium – hence the significantly higher incidence of fractures in women over 50 years of age.

A diet rich in calcium and vitamin D is essential to maintain bone density. Milk, cheese and yoghurt are rich sources of calcium. Vitamin D is found in butter, fish, meat and sunlight. In addition regular exercise is important to aid circulation to muscles, joints and bones to prevent symptoms of rheumatism and the development of a 'dowager's hump' in later life.

Skin changes

Some drying and wrinkling may occur. Attention to diet, general good health, regular exercise, relaxation, and use of skin preparations will help to maintain skin texture. Smoking and heavy drinking should be discouraged.

Breast changes

Some changes occur, including some shrinkage of breast tissue. A well-fitting bra will give support.

Shrinkage of vaginal and vulval tissue

This occurs as a result of decreasing oestrogen levels. If a couple enjoy an active sex life, the woman is less likely to suffer vaginal symptoms. Some women suffer loss of libido around the menopause. General health measures and appropriate medical treatment will help to alleviate any distressing symptoms. Sexual desire need not be affected.

THE WELL WOMAN CLINIC

Women of all ages should receive regular 'Well Woman' checks but this is particularly important during the peri-menopausal years. A physical check up will be given, including weight and blood pressure checks. A sample of urine will be tested.

BREAST AWARENESS

Every woman should be aware of the normal shape and consistency of her breast tissue, remembering that it extends into the armpit area. During the menstrual cycle a woman's breasts naturally fluctuate in size and sometimes in tenderness. Any lumps or unusual symptoms which persist should be reported to a doctor or practice nurse. Women should be aware that breast cancer can develop at any time and early diagnosis is of vital importance. Breast awareness is especially important during the peri-menopausal years.

CERVICAL SMEAR

This simple test is used to detect early changes that occur in the cervix before cancer develops. If abnormal cells are found sufficiently early, cancer may be prevented. All women should have regular cervical smears as frequently as medically advised.

DIET AND EXERCISE

A healthy diet should include sufficient fibre to give added bulk without extra calories and to maintain a regular bowel habit. Carbohydrate consumption should be low, avoiding sweet sugary foods. The diet should include plenty of fish, cheese, milk (preferably skimmed), yoghurt, green vegetables, wholemeal bread and muesli.

Certain vitamin preparations are helpful in relieving symptoms such as hot flushes, tiredness and mild depression. Vitamin B6 is available as tablets, but it also occurs naturally in yeast, wheat-germ, bananas, chicken and meat. Vitamin E is also helpful in reducing the number and severity of hot flushes. It occurs naturally in wheat-germ and sunflower oil and can also be taken in tablet form.

Exercise, preferably outdoor, should be included as part of daily life. Exercise in any form helps increase the blood supply to the muscles, joints, and bones, to maintain fitness and encourage a sense of well-being. There is a clear relationship between a healthy body and an easier menopause.

HORMONE REPLACEMENT THERAPY (HRT)

If symptoms, such as frequent disabling hot flushes or vaginitis, are severe, a doctor may prescribe natural oestrogen with progestogen usually in the form of tablets. The content of oestrogen in these pills is very much lower than the dose of synthetic oestrogen in the contraceptive pill. When hormone replacement therapy is taken, there is less anxiety about the risks of heart disease and cancer. A positive benefit of HRT is in the prevention of osteoporosis, a serious and frequently disabling condition. All women should discuss the indications for HRT with their doctors. There are various ways of taking HRT:

- Tablets taken daily by mouth.
- Patches applied to the skin and changed every few days.
- Hormone implants or pellets inserted under the skin, and replaced every few months.

■ HRT cream or pessaries if vaginal dryness is the main problem.

The majority of women will go through the menopause with very little difficulty, and will emerge somewhat enriched, more mature, and with a new sexual freedom. The absence of monthly periods and the knowledge that there is no possibility of pregnancy will be welcomed.

DECLINING FERTILITY DURING THE PRE-MENOPAUSE

The pre-menopause may last for as long as 10 years for some women, from 45–55 years of age, for example. For other women it may only take two years from start to finish. The length of the pre-menopause and the severity of associated symptoms varies considerably from woman to woman. Fertility may disappear then reappear months later. It is impossible to predict when fertility will end, although a woman's pattern may be similar to that of her mother or sisters.

Besides the physical and psychological problems of the pre-menopause there is the additional problem of family planning. Many women fear the 'menopausal baby', with the well-documented increased risk of Down's Syndrome. In addition, there may be psychological problems created for the parents at a time in life when their offspring may be grown up and they feel unable to cope with an unplanned pregnancy. This fear may lead to reluctance to have sexual intercourse. As cycles become irregular, each month brings anxiety and this is increased when a period is missed.

REPRODUCTIVE POTENTIAL IN THE OLDER WOMAN

All women should realise that they become less fertile as they grow older. In countries where there is no family planning, the average time between the birth of the last child and the menopause is 12 years.

Dr Evelyn Billings quotes these figures for women where no birth control method is used.

■ In the age group 40–45 years, less than 35 per cent of women are still fertile.
■ In the age group 45–50 years, less than one per cent of women are still fertile.
■ Over 50 years, pregnancy is rare.

FERTILITY AWARENESS DURING THE PRE-MENOPAUSE

If a woman has previous experience of fertility awareness during normal fertile cycles this can be very helpful in identifying early changes related to the pre-menopause. It is possible to start using natural family planning at this time despite cyclic irregularities, provided a woman has the support of an experienced NFP teacher. Women who have used natural methods successfully for a number of years will need further help to interpret their charts as cycles become irregular.

CYCLIC CHANGES

It is important that women are aware of the possible cyclic variations leading up to the menopause. As fertility progressively declines, ovulation tends to become irregular and infrequent with subsequent irregularity of menstruation. There may be variations in cycle length both pre- and post-ovulatory, the presence or absence of ovulation, or shortening of the luteal phase. The temperature shift will vary accordingly. Menstrual loss will vary from scant to very heavy bleeding which could result in anaemia and fatigue. The cervical mucus diminishes in quantity and loses its fertile characteristics in many cycles. A typical pattern of infertility will be recognised – persistent dry days are most common, but other women will have persistent moistness, an unchanging pattern of secretions.

VARIATIONS IN CYCLE LENGTH
- Average length cycles.
- Shorter cycles than usual (23 days or less).
- Very long cycles.

OVULATORY CYCLES
- Ovulation may occur early resulting in an early temperature shift.
- Ovulation may be delayed resulting in a delayed temperature shift.
- Shortened post-ovulatory or luteal phases (8–10 days or less).
- Menstrual loss will be varied.

ANOVULATORY CYCLES
- Monophasic cycles shown by the absence of a temperature shift.
- Varied length – often persistent dryness throughout.
- Bleeding is normally very light.

EFFECTS ON MUCUS PATTERN
- Persistent dryness is most common.
- A basic infertile pattern (BIP) of moistness – constant, unchanging pattern for at least 2 weeks.
- Increasing numbers of dry days as mucus production decreases.
- Occasional sticky mucus patches during otherwise dry days.
- Decreasing amounts of slippery stretchy mucus.
- Mucus pattern starting very early.
- Very short mucus build-up prior to temperature shift.

EFFECTS ON TEMPERATURE
- Variations in shift day dependent on cycle length and length of pre- and post-ovulatory phases.
- Monophasic chart in anovulatory cycles.

CHANGES IN VAGINAL BLEEDING

There may be variations in the amount and regularity of menstrual loss:

- Heavy prolonged bleeding with clots.
- Sudden brief or more prolonged episodes of bleeding or flooding.
- Bleeding may be very light.
- Spotting may occur either between periods or in place of a true period.

RECOGNISING A TRUE PERIOD

- A true period follows ovulation. It is preceded by a temperature shift 10–14 days earlier.
- Any other bleeding may be associated with oestrogen activity, and increased fertility.

Important note: If periods are getting further apart, shorter and lighter then there is generally no cause for concern. But if periods are getting closer together, longer and heavier, or if there is any bleeding between periods, medical advice must be sought. Menstrual disturbance may be due to hormone imbalance, but it should always be investigated as there are many other causes. Any woman who experiences vaginal bleeding more than one year after her last menstruation should seek medical advice.

RECOGNISING SIGNS OF INFERTILITY

As fertility declines during the pre-menopausal years, the key to successful use of natural methods lies not so much in identifying fertility but in positively identifying the increasingly lengthy periods of infertility.

MUCUS SYMPTOM

- Dryness – there may be long periods of dryness.
- Basic infertile pattern – continuous unchanging pattern of moistness. Some women will experience an unchanging pattern of secretions, which may be seen as a pasty white discharge forming the basic infertile pattern. It may be helpful to check the secretions using the 'glass of water test'. Non-fertile secretions, often comprising moisture and vaginal cells, will disperse. Fertile mucus secretions, of cervical origin, form a blob or string.

CERVIX

The cervix will be low, firm, closed and tilted.

TEMPERATURE

The pattern will be monophasic (on one level, indicating absence of ovulation).

RECORDING ON THE PRE-MENOPAUSAL CHART

The special 16 week pre-menopausal chart should be used to record daily observations of fertility indicators and also information about general health, and pre-menopausal symptoms. The extended chart makes it easier to monitor cyclic variability over a period of four months.

BLEEDING AND MUCUS SYMPTOM

■ Days of a period or blood loss are marked with a **P.** Indicate amount of bleeding, for example spotting/light/moderate/heavy bleeding.
■ Days when there is a dry sensation and no visible mucus are marked with a **D.**
■ Moist days forming the basic infertile pattern (BIP) should be marked with an **m.**
■ Day of sticky white/creamy mucus are marked with an **M.**
■ Any days of highly fertile transparent, slippery, stretchy mucus are marked with an **F.**

CERVICAL CHANGES

These may give the earliest information about approaching fertility.
The infertile cervix is represented by:
■ A solid black circle showing it to be firm and closed.

■ The symbol being placed on the baseline showing it to be low.
■ A diagonal line showing the tilt.
The fertile cervix is represented by:
■ An open circle showing softening.
■ An inner ring showing that the os is open.
■ The symbol being placed higher in the space provided to show elevated position.
■ A vertical line below to show the straight position.

TEMPERATURE

■ The daily waking temperature should be recorded throughout the cycle.
■ It is important to record at least six low temperatures.

OTHER SYMPTOMS

Record hot flushes and other symptoms of the pre-menopause, physical and emotional changes and any other disturbances.

USE OF COLOUR

The red/yellow/green colour code can be added as part of the chart interpretation highlighting the phases of fertility and infertility, and indicating the times available for intercourse.

Fig 13.1 Pre-menopausal chart. The pattern of fertility and infertility is shown by a correlation between the temperature mucus and cervical signs. Intercourse is restricted to the infertile phases indicated by the pre-menopausal guidelines. Note the recording of hot flushes and other personal notes.

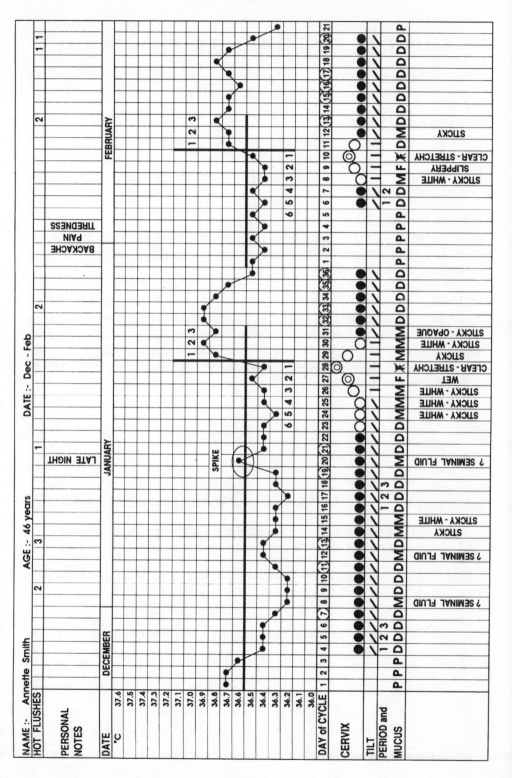

RECOGNISING SIGNS WHICH MAY INDICATE FERTILITY

TEMPERATURE
The temperature pattern will be biphasic, confirming ovulation.

PERIOD OR BLEEDING
Any bleeding must be regarded as potentially fertile because:
- Bleeding may be associated with ovulation.
- Bleeding identified as a true period could mask the mucus symptom in a very short cycle.

MUCUS SYMPTOM
- If BIP is of dry days, then any change from dryness indicates fertility.
- If BIP is of moistness, then any change from the established infertile pattern indicates fertility.

CERVIX
The first change from the infertile cervix indicates fertility. Many pre-menopausal women find the earliest information about times of fertility and infertility is shown by the cervix. The earliest sign of change from the infertile pattern may indicate approaching fertility. This may be shown by either the cervix or the mucus.

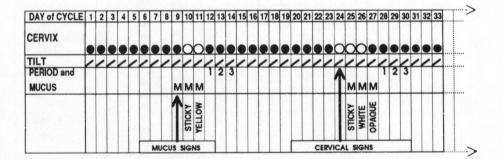

Fig. 13.2 Recording the earliest sign of fertility. The arrows indicate the earliest sign of fertility shown either by the first mucus signs or the first change in the cervix, whichever comes first.

GUIDELINES TO AVOID PREGNANCY DURING THE PRE-MENOPAUSE

Use the coverline technique to identify the temperature shift.

Pre-ovulatory phases, and anovulatory cycles

Bleeding
■ Any day of blood loss could mask early mucus symptoms in a short cycle.

Mucus symptom
■ Dry days are infertile – any change from dryness could indicate approaching fertility.
■ BIP of moistness – any change from BIP could indicate approaching fertility.

Cervical signs
■ Days on which the cervix is low, firm, closed and tilted are infertile.
■ Any change from the infertile state could indicate approaching fertility.

It is advisable to double check mucus and cervical signs to minimise errors of interpretation.

■ **The S minus 20 rule or Doering rule can no longer be used as a double check.**

■ Intercourse should be restricted to alternate evenings during the infertile pattern to allow time for observation during the day, and to avoid confusion with seminal fluid.

■ Intercourse should be avoided during any bleeding and for the following three days.

■ Intercourse should be avoided at the first sign of fertility while the fertile signs last, and for three days after return to the infertile pattern. This allows time to ensure that the BIP is re-established and that fertile signs are not leading to ovulation.

Post-ovulatory phases
■ Intercourse can be resumed after the third high temperature past peak day.

In cycles where the temperature shift occurs confirming ovulation, intercourse can be resumed without restrictions until the onset of the next period.

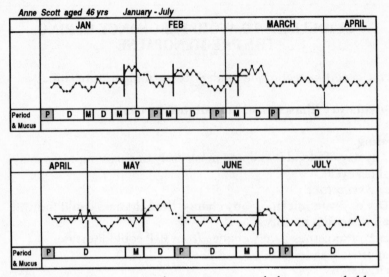

Fig 13.3 *Two consecutive 16 week pre-menopausal charts recorded by a 46 year old woman. Note the irregularity of the cycles. Using an extended coverline, some cycles are biphasic and others are monophasic.*

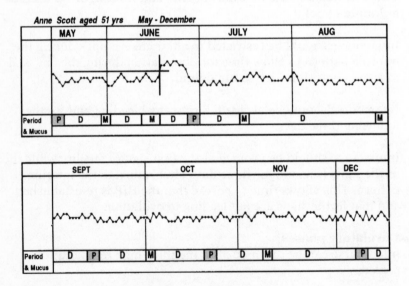

Fig 13.4 *Post-menopausal infertility. Five years later there is only evidence of ovulation once, in June. Following this there are six months without further signs of ovulation. There are periods of blood loss, but very little mucus. As this woman is over 50 with six anovular cycles, she will no longer be fertile, so can stop charting.*

EFFECTIVENESS DURING THE PRE-MENOPAUSE

If a couple choose to restrict intercourse until the post-ovulatory phase is confirmed, there is almost no chance of pregnancy, but there may be very long periods of abstinence and this can put strains on the relationship. A woman who is experienced in observing mucus and cervical signs may choose to use the pre-ovulatory phase for intercourse in addition, therefore increasing the time available for intercourse. Although it should be understood that there is always a slight risk of pregnancy in the pre-ovulatory phase, this is small, but couples should have the opportunity to consider all their options and to consider the effects on their relationship. Most couples who understand their fertility will be reassured by observing signs of declining fertility and can be helped to feel confident in using natural methods at this time.

14. Infertility and Subfertility

DEFINING FERTILITY PROBLEMS

An infertile couple is a couple who are unable to conceive after one year of regular intercourse. (Sterility is a term reserved for a couple who can never conceive.) Subfertility denotes a reduced state of fertility, whereby some factors such as a low sperm count or damaged fallopian tubes may reduce the chances of conception.

It is now estimated that one in six couples have fertility problems. The peak of fertility for both men and women occurs around 17–28 years. Many couples are now postponing childbearing until later in life, for career or social reasons. More than 50 per cent of women over 35 years will take up to two years to conceive their first child. Even when a couple of normal fertility have intercourse at the most fertile time in the cycle, it takes an average of three cycles for conception to occur. From all this it will be apparent that most couples presenting with fertility problems will eventually become pregnant without treatment.

FACTORS INVOLVED IN CONCEPTION

If conception is to occur, the most important physiological conditions required are that a woman must ovulate, her fallopian tubes must be patent and her partner should have an adequate number of live, normal sperm capable of penetrating her fertile cervical mucus and subsequently meeting the ovum. Any couple planning a pregnancy should be in good health, but this is especially important for a couple with fertility problems.

PRE-CONCEPTUAL CARE

The great majority of couples planning pregnancy will conceive without problems, the mother will have a normal pregnancy and the birth of the baby will be straightforward. For couples with fertility problems, there are many advantages in improving good general health in the pre-conceptual period, to provide optimum conditions for conception and pregnancy.

Both partners should enjoy a well-balanced diet, avoiding excessive amounts of fatty foods or sugars, and eating plenty of fresh fruit, whole grain foods, and vegetables. Maintenance of an optimum weight for height is important. Any woman who is either very underweight or overweight may have difficulties in conceiving. Alcohol should be reduced to a minimum or given up, as in excess it can seriously affect the developing foetus. Smoking should likewise be stopped prior to conception because it reduces the oxygen supply to the developing foetus and may result in a baby of low birth weight and poor health. The incidence of miscarriages is also significantly higher in women who smoke.

It is a wise precaution to avoid all drugs in the pre-conception period, and during pregnancy and breast-feeding. Only medication prescribed by a doctor, who is aware of the planned pregnancy, should be taken. Adequate rest and sleep are important. Undue fatigue and stress should be avoided. It may be a good time to learn a relaxation technique that will be beneficial during pregnancy, childbirth and in the later years. Daily exercise is important to promote a sense of well-being and maintain fitness, but excessive exercising should be avoided as it may cause weight loss and hormone imbalance, and could inhibit ovulation. It is important that a couple enjoy sex and do not become too preoccupied with plans for conception. If sex is pleasurable for both partners, then it is likely to be more frequent and the relationship will be enhanced.

Whenever possible a couple should discuss with their doctor their intentions to plan a pregnancy. The opportunity may arise naturally if a method of contraception is stopped in order to achieve pregnancy, for example if an IUD is removed. But by the nature of natural family planning, there may be no such apparent opportunity for discussion with a doctor. The most essential aspect of pre-conceptual care is to ensure that a woman is immune to rubella (German measles). If the developing foetus is exposed to the rubella virus in the first 12 weeks, there may be serious effects including blindness, deafness and mental retardation. This can be avoided by a simple blood test to detect rubella antibodies in the mother's blood, and then immunisation if necessary.

Pre-conceptual care is very important for those couples who have experienced miscarriages, complications of pregnancy, or sadly, have lost a child. A family history of congenital disease or deformity is a strong indication for pre-conceptual care. The importance of vitamin B in the prevention of spina-bifida has been established. It is recommended that all women considering pregnancy should take folic acid.

THE CAUSE OF FERTILITY PROBLEMS

Infertility may be caused by problems in either partner or both. An estimated 40 per cent of infertility cases are found to be related to the woman, a further 40 per cent are found to originate in the man, 10 per cent of cases are caused by low fertility in both partners and in the remaining 10 per cent no cause will be found. It is important that even when the major cause of infertility rests with one partner, the problem should be viewed as the problem of the couple rather than of an individual.

Many women delay childbearing until their late 20s or early 30s. A woman is at her most fertile between 17 and 28 years, when cycles are more consistently regular and ovulatory. If fertility problems first present when a women is 35, instead of 25, it can be more difficult to treat because of the natural decline in fertility. The man's age is not a significant factor.

MALE INFERTILITY

The male partner may be infertile or subfertile as a result of the following factors:

- Sperm production may be impaired by occupational hazards. This must be considered for men who work with chemicals, atomic energy, radiation or in conditions of excessive heat.
- To avoid over-heating of the testes, men should avoid wearing tight underpants and jeans.
- General ill health, fatigue and stress may cause temporary infertility.
- Sexually transmitted diseases, including chlamydia, gonorrhoea and non-specific urethritis.
- Orchitis or inflammation of the testes which may occur as a complication of mumps contracted after puberty.
- Congenital abnormalities of the reproductive tract, or abnormalities in the male sex hormone or pituitary hormone systems.
- Certain drugs may reduce libido (sexual desire), and potency (virility), and may therefore affect fertility, such as tranquillisers and some drugs used to treat high blood pressure.
- Drugs used in the treatment of cancer may affect the testes and impair sperm production.
- Psychological pressures may lead to sexual problems including impotence (failure to achieve or maintain an erection), and severe premature ejaculation. Psycho-sexual counselling may be required.

FEMALE INFERTILITY

There are a number of causes of infertility or subfertility in the female partner.
Tubal damage accounts for about one third of all cases of female infertility.
Pelvic inflammatory disease (PID) – the microscopic hairs lining the tubes are easily damaged by any pelvic infection. PID may occur following childbirth, abortion, sexually transmitted diseases, particularly chlamydia, or following insertion of an intrauterine device. This tubal damage impedes the passage of the sperm and the ovum making conception unlikely.
Adhesions – these are bands of fibrous tissue in the pelvis that may develop after surgery, or following pelvic infection. They may prevent the release of the ovum or impede its passage to or within the tube.
Ectopic pregnancy – if conception occurs, the fertilised ovum may be unable to pass along the damaged tube, which may have very poor muscular movement. The embryo will continue to develop in the tube, resulting in a tubal or ectopic pregnancy. If this is undiagnosed, rupture of the tube may follow. A woman who has an ectopic pregnancy will complain of severe one-sided abdominal pain which may be accompanied by vaginal bleeding. This condition requires immediate surgical intervention.
Surgical sterilisation – some women who have previously been sterilised may wish to regain their fertility (for example following remarriage or the

death of a child). The extent of tubal damage incurred at the time of sterilisation will determine the chances of successful reversal.

Hormonal imbalance – imbalance of the female sex hormone or pituitary
hormone systems may be responsible for infertility. Excessive weight loss or
anorexia nervosa may cause anovulation and secondary amenorrhoea.

Unruptured follicle syndrome – very rarely a follicle may mature in the
ovary, but then for some reason fail to rupture and release the ovum. A corpus luteum will form and produce progesterone. This is the luteinised
unruptured follicle syndrome (LUF). Although this will be an anovulatory
cycle, the temperature chart will be biphasic and may have a longer luteal
phase than normal.

Endometriosis – this is a condition where endometrial tissue grows in
abnormal places such as on the surface of the ovaries, or within the fallopian tubes. It may prevent passage of the ovum from the ovary to the tube,
or impede passage of the sperm or ovum within the tube. Endometriosis
may be suspected if a woman develops pain at ovulation, before or during
menstruation, or complains of discomfort during intercourse. A dark brown
(chocolate) discharge is characteristic of endometriosis.

Fibroids – these are abnormal growths of muscular tissue in the uterus
which may block the tubes or impair implantation resulting in early miscarriage. Fibroids may cause heavy or painful periods.

Damaged cervix – any operative treatment of the cervix may damage the
mucus membrane lining the cervical canal and so interfere with cervical
mucus production.

Drugs may impair production of cervical mucus. These include antihista-
mines used to dry up the secretions in a common cold, or for hay fever, or
other allergic conditions, and anti-inflammatory drugs used in the treatment of rheumatism.

Stress – the effect of stress on the menstrual cycle has already been discussed. A common reaction to stress is to delay ovulation. The mucus
build-up will be interrupted and the temperature shift will likewise be
delayed, resulting in a long cycle. Severe stress may completely suppress
ovulation, resulting in anovulatory cycles and subsequent infertility.
Increasing anxiety and the stress of infertility investigations may exacerbate
the problem.

Idiopathic infertility – this is a term used to describe a situation in which
there is no apparent cause of infertility. After thorough investigation, about
10 per cent of infertile couples will be told that with the present state of
knowledge there is no specific reason to explain their infertility.

MISCARRIAGES

Miscarriage or spontaneous abortion occurs most commonly around 10–14
weeks of pregnancy.

Care should be taken in the early months of pregnancy to avoid strenu-
ous or abnormal activity. It is wise to avoid intercourse at times when the

period is due in the first three months. During pregnancy, unless a couple are medically advised otherwise, intercourse can take place as desired provided a woman feels comfortable.

There are many causes of miscarriage:
■ Abnormality of the foetus.
■ Incompetent cervix, a term used to describe a cervix which is unable to provide sufficient support for pregnancy to continue beyond about 12–16 weeks, and may therefore be a cause of recurrent miscarriages.
■ Other abnormalities of the genital tract such as fibroids.
■ Hormone imbalance.

Often the reason for the miscarriage is not diagnosed. The miscarriage may be complete or incomplete. In the latter case a dilatation and curettage (D&C) will be performed to remove any retained products of conception. A pelvic examination is carried out about six weeks after a miscarriage, and normal physiology returns by three months. For many couples, miscarriage is a traumatic experience physically and psychologically. It is wise to wait for this time before planning a further pregnancy to allow time for recovery and readjustment.

KERRY AND IAN: Kerry, aged 30, had a two-year-old son, but had been trying to conceive for the past year. She complained of heavy delayed periods, which her consultant gynaecologist diagnosed as early miscarriages. This caused the couple very considerable distress. Following sympto-thermal charting, it became apparent that Kerry had very delayed ovulations. They had previously been timing intercourse around day 14, the day they thought was the most fertile time. By learning to recognise her mucus symptom, Kerry realised that her fertile phase was much later, and conceived following intercourse on day 23, the day before peak day.

VALUE OF FERTILITY AWARENESS

Many couples have difficulty conceiving when there is no serious physical problem to account for their reduced fertility. Fertility awareness can be a very valuable means of optimising the chances of pregnancy. Many couples remain ignorant about their fertility, and for some education may be all that is required to achieve conception.

Ideally couples should learn about fertility before they are referred to a hospital fertility clinic. As the woman learns to keep accurate records of her fertility cycles on the sympto-thermal chart, any variation from the normal will be apparent. The sympto-thermal chart is a diagnostic aid which can give the following information:

TEMPERATURE READINGS

- A monophasic chart shows that there has been no ovulation.
- A biphasic chart with a short luteal phase (less than nine days) is significant – fertilisation may occur but there is insufficient time for implantation.
- The short cycle showing early ovulation, or the long cycle showing late ovulation, may highlight the mis-timing of intercourse. This commonly occurs with women who have been told that they should have intercourse on the 14th day or mid-cycle.

OBSERVATION OF CERVICAL MUCUS

- Days of maximum fertility are recognised by the presence of slippery, transparent, stretchy mucus. These days occur immediately prior to ovulation and precede the temperature shift. There may be irregular cycles or fertile mucus signs may last only 24–48 hours. This mucus symptom provides the most accurate means of timing intercourse to optimise the chances of conception.

DIANE AND TED: Diane and Ted had been trying for a baby for four years. They had been fully investigated at the fertility clinic, where there was said to be no apparent cause for infertility. Although a highly educated couple, they had very little understanding of their own physiology. At the first interview, it became apparent that Diane had irregular cycles (25–33 days). A hectic lifestyle, including pressures at work, resulted in infrequent intercourse. Increasing fertility awareness allowed Diane to experience the sensation of a very short mucus build-up, and time intercourse appropriately. She conceived in her second cycle of charting.

HOME-KITS TO PREDICT OVULATION

The day before ovulation there is normally a sudden surge of luteinising hormone (LH), which can be identified in simple home tests. Clearplan One-Step is one such test in which a dipstick is held in a stream of urine first thing in the morning. A positive LH test shows a blue line after five minutes. First Response is a similar urine test, which identifies the LH surge by means of an easy-to-read colour change.

Tests are carried out for between five and 10 days of the cycle, dependent on cycle length and regularity. They indicate the time of maximum fertility. As most women will ovulate within 12–24 hours of the positive test, intercourse during this time carries the highest chance of pregnancy. Home kits are relatively expensive, but can be a valuable aid for women experiencing difficulty observing the mucus symptom.

SIGNS INDICATING POSSIBLE CAUSES OF INFERTILITY

■ Monophasic charts.
■ Luteal phases of 10 days or less.
■ Absence of fertile mucus.

If any of these signs recur on three consecutive cycles, the woman should be referred for further investigations. Some fertility investigations may be carried out in general practice. The doctor will then discuss with the couple the possibility of referral for consultant advice.

THE FERTILITY CLINIC

MEDICAL HISTORY

A couple will usually be seen together initially, then both partners may be seen individually, when personal questions can be asked to establish previous sexual history, including any past history of sexually transmitted disease of which the partner may be unaware. A woman will be asked about previous pregnancies including abortions, and a man may be asked about any previous children he believes he has fathered. These details form a vital part of the infertility investigations, and are treated with the strictest confidence throughout.

INVESTIGATION OF MALE INFERTILITY

A physical examination will be carried out to exclude any apparent infections or abnormalities, and a specimen of seminal fluid will be analysed. A man's sperm count may vary from time to time, and so a number of tests should be carried out. If these semen analyses show sperm of consistently poor quality or quantity, then further investigations will be required to determine the cause of the problem.

NORMAL SPERM COUNT

Volume	1 – 6 ml
Count	> 20 million per ml
Abnormal forms	<30 per cent
No bacteria seen	

TREATMENT OF MALE INFERTILITY

This is still in its infancy and at present is relatively ineffective. Treatment with male hormones is being tried, but with little success. If the man is found to have a low sperm count, artificial insemination may be offered. The man's sperm will be used wherever possible (this is known as AIH – Artificial insemination by husband) and injected directly into the uterus during the fertile phase of the cycle. Some of the more recent techniques of assisted conception are able to optimise the chances of fertilisation using a very low number of sperm with some success.

Some men may seek help to restore their fertility following surgical sterilisation (vasectomy). Although surgical reversal may appear successful, the presence of anti-sperm antibodies may prevent the return of fertility. Where it is not possible to use the partner's sperm donor insemination (AID) may be offered.

INVESTIGATION OF FEMALE INFERTILITY
A physical and gynaecological examination will be done to exclude obvious abnormalities and infections. This will include a vaginal examination.

Blood tests
Blood tests may be done to measure female sex hormones, and pituitary hormone levels.

Sex hormones – oestrogen and progesterone levels are measured. The progesterone levels are estimated in the mid-luteal phase (Day 21 progesterone) to give an indication as to whether ovulation has occurred and whether the corpus luteum is producing sufficient progesterone to sustain pregnancy. Understanding fertility awareness can assist in the accurate timing of this test.

Pituitary hormones – follicle stimulating hormone, and luteinising hormone levels will be checked. Prolactin levels will also be measured. An excess of prolactin will block ovulation (compare the effect during breastfeeding).

Cervical mucus tests
A specimen of cervical mucus is taken at the appropriate time to estimate its fertile characteristics. The amount, the appearance and the texture of the mucus, including the Spinnbarkeit test, and the ferning effect produced by fertile mucus are checked. A specimen of fertile cervical mucus is taken post-coitally, to determine sperm/mucus compatibility. If a woman is able to recognise fertile mucus, she will know the best time for this test to be carried out.

Laparoscopy
This is a technique used to view the ovaries, tubes and uterus, by an instrument known as a laparoscope. Laparoscopy involves two incisions, one just below the umbilicus and the other on the pubic hair line. This allows the organs to be manipulated into view. While the fallopian tubes are in view, a dye may be passed through the cervix to check for blockages in the tubes. If the tubes are patent, the dye will be seen to pass into the abdominal cavity. Fibroids, adhesions, endometriosis and tubal damage may all be diagnosed by laparoscopy.

Ultrasound scanning
Ultrasound scanning can be used as an aid to diagnosing the cause of infertility. A scan will reveal the size and position of the uterus, tubes and ovaries. It will also show the thickness of the endometrium and any uterine

fibroids or ovarian cysts. The scan may be used to monitor the growth and maturation of ovarian follicles, and to observe ovulation. If conception occurs, a scan will assist in the diagnosis of early pregnancy, and can be used to monitor the development of the unborn child.

TREATMENT OF FEMALE INFERTILITY

Hormonal treatment
If ovulation is not occurring, fertility drugs such as clomiphene are frequently successful in inducing ovulation and subsequent pregnancy, but the side effects must be borne in mind. The phenomenon of multiple births following the use of fertility drugs is widely known, although this is less common with the newer drugs and careful monitoring of the dosage.

Tubal surgery
Tubal surgery aims to restore the function of the fallopian tubes. Where blockage is caused by adhesions outside the tubes, the treatment is very successful, but when the tubal lining is damaged, the success rate is much lower in spite of new surgical techniques, including laser treatment and the use of specially-designed microscopes.

In-vitro fertilisation
In vitro (in glass) fertilisation is used as a means of by-passing blocked or damaged tubes. The treatment involves careful monitoring of the cycle to determine the time of ovulation Fertility drugs are used to ensure that several ova will reach maturity, at which time they can be retrieved. A fresh sample of the husband's sperm is then placed with the ova in a petri-dish and observed. If fertilisation is successful, the embryos are grown for about three days, at which time they will be transferred via a catheter through the cervix high up into the uterus.

The stimulation of several ova to maturity is necessary in an attempt to achieve at least three embryos – the optimum number required to achieve successful implantation and the maximum chance of pregnancy. It is rare for all three embryos to implant successfully. IVF programmes are costly in terms of time and money. The success rate is variable, but is seldom higher than 30 per cent. It is also costly in human terms, as the procedure can be very stressful for a couple. Specialist fertility counselling should be available.

EMOTIONAL EFFECTS OF INFERTILITY ON A COUPLE

Couples who are faced with fertility problems may experience a series of emotional reactions. For some these may be as hard to cope with as the feeling of loss following a bereavement. Such couples should know that they share a common experience with many others. One couple in six experiences fertility problems, but the number remaining childless is small.

The first reaction may be one of surprise when pregnancy does not follow as planned after birth control measures are stopped. The couple may deny their disappointment both to themselves and to others, and consequently are likely to delay in seeking help. Some couples find their unhappiness increased by well meaning relatives and friends whether they commiserate on their failure to conceive or pressurise them by offering them kind but inappropriate advice. Other couples can feel isolated as their friends have children. If one partner longs for a child more than the other, this can produce tension in the relationship.

Medical advice will provide the solution for many couples. As investigations lead to diagnosis, and treatment eases the way to pregnancy, previous anxieties will be forgotten. For others stress and tension may be increased as they face long waits for hospital appointments, test results, and treatment. Fertility problems inevitably create anxiety, and it should be realised that stress can in turn contribute to the delay in conception. Fertility counselling can be very helpful at this time, and if the general practitioner and practice nurse are also aware of such problems they can give valuable support.

15. Contraception, Sterilisation and Abortion

CONTRACEPTION

This section on contraception is included to give factual information about other methods of birth control, and to have regard to factors which may affect the future fertility of a couple if they subsequently wish to have a child.

FAMILY PLANNING ADVICE
At the first visit there should be adequate time available for counselling. Psychological and emotional factors, and ethical matters relative to the couple need to be considered with sensitivity. These should be reflected in the way couples are helped to choose a method. Time is needed to give information and education. A couple who have learnt fertility awareness will be in a better position to understand not only how the method works, but the effectiveness, the advantages and the possible disadvantages.

Family planning method	Range of failure rates
Combined pill	<1–3+
Progestogen-only pill	1–4+
Injectables and implants	<1-2
Intra-uterine system (IUS)	<1
Intra-uterine device (IUD)	<1–2
Diaphragm or cap with spermicide	4–18
Condom (male and female)	2–15
NFP – Sympto-thermal	2–15

Sterilisation	
Male sterilisation or vasectomy	0.1
Female sterilisation	0.5

Table 15.1 Comparison of failure rates for different methods per 100 woman years (FPA 1995)

Many teenagers risk pregnancy rather than seek advice about family planning. They need reassurance that their confidentiality will be respected. Young people may be anxious and looking for information and advice about sexually transmitted infections and HIV. It is important that they should not feel pressurised and should be able to discuss the advantages –

both physical and psychological – of postponing sex. They need sympathetic counselling in confidence to minimise the risks of damaging future fertility and to reduce the risk of unintended pregnancy.

In considering the effectiveness of family planning, the practical or user failure is the most significant factor. This can be measured by the number of unplanned pregnancies per 100 woman years. Where two figures are quoted, the first figure denotes careful or consistent use and the second figure denotes less careful or inconsistent use of the method. For example, with careful and consistent use the condom has a failure rate around 2 per cent but with less careful and inconsistent use, the failure rate could be as high as 15 per cent. Not all methods have a user failure rate, for example implants, injectables and IUD's have a very low failure rate and this is always due to method failure.

HORMONAL CONTRACEPTION

All methods of hormonal contraception act by altering the normal reproductive physiology of a woman's body. In this category there are five methods of contraception to be considered.

- Combined pill
- Progestogen-only pill
- Injectables
- Implants
- Intra-uterine system

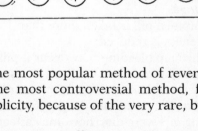

*Fig 15.1 Combined pills –
taken 21 days out of 28*

THE COMBINED PILL

The contraceptive pill remains the most popular method of reversible contraception. It is possibly also the most controversial method, frequently receiving widespread adverse publicity, because of the very rare, but serious or even fatal side effects.

For normal healthy young women, it is efficient and has many advantages, but careful screening is essential. Factors such as severe migraine, obesity and heavy smoking are contra-indications to pill use. A family history of cardio-vascular disease, occurring at a younger age (less than 45 years), breast cancer and diabetes for example, will be taken into consideration.

The combined pill contains two hormones – synthetic oestrogen and progestogen – and is taken daily, usually for 21 days out of 28.

Action

The combined pill acts by suppressing the sex hormone system, which normally controls the menstrual cycle, thus blocking the process leading to ovulation. It does this in three ways:

■ FSH is reduced, preventing the development and maturation of ovarian follicles.
■ The LH surge is stopped, so the ovum is not released.
■ The progestogen component of the combined pill prevents sperm from entering the uterus by stimulating the production of thick barrier-type mucus.

As the normal menstrual cycle is suppressed, periods will be replaced by a hormone withdrawal bleed a few days after the pills are stopped. Withdrawal bleeds are usually less painful and lighter than normal menstrual periods.

Effectiveness

With careful use, less than one woman in 100 will get pregnant in a year. With less careful use, three or more women will get pregnant in a year.

Advantages

■ Provided the pills are taken as directed, it is an extremely effective method.
■ It may relieve anxiety about unplanned pregnancy.
■ It allows spontaneous intercourse throughout the cycle.
■ Periods are usually shorter, lighter and less painful.
■ Symptoms of pre-menstrual syndrome may be relieved.
■ There is good evidence that the pill protects against endometrial and ovarian cancer.

Disadvantages

■ If a combined pill is taken more than 12 hours late, the contraceptive effectiveness is reduced.
■ Breakthrough bleeding may occur if pills are missed.
■ Any woman prescribed medication, especially antibiotics, or drugs for epilepsy should ensure that her doctor knows that she is taking the contraceptive pill, as certain drugs affect its efficacy.
■ Vomiting or severe diarrhoea may affect the absorption of the pill.
■ For a few women, the return of fertility may be delayed after stopping the pill.

Minor side effects

Side effects commonly occur, particularly during the first few cycles of pill-taking, as the body adjusts to the increased level of hormones. Some of these effects are similar to those experienced in the early weeks of pregnancy, such as nausea, breast tenderness, bloating, headaches, and should disappear after the first two or three cycles. Although side effects are frequently considered of nuisance value only, nevertheless if they are causing concern a woman should seek advice.

Major complications
Cardiovascular disease
Women taking the pill should be alert to the possible warning signs of thrombosis. These include severe pain in the calf of one leg, severe pains in the chest and unexplained breathlessness or cough with blood-stained sputum.

Cancer of the cervix
There is some anxiety about increased risk of cancer of the cervix. Among women who have taken the pill for more than five years, there is an increase in the number of abnormal cervical smears. This may also be related to sexual behaviour or a sexually transmitted virus, or to smoking. It is important for all women to have their regular cervical smears.

Breast cancer
There is some research suggesting that taking the combined pill when young, and pill-taking for several years may slightly increase the risk of unusually early breast cancer (before 35 years of age). Further research is underway to clarify this.

THE PROGESTOGEN-ONLY PILL
The progestogen-only pill is taken every day without a break. It has fewer associated side effects, but shows a higher failure rate than the combined pills.

Action
The progestogen-only pill acts by:
- Altering the cervical mucus. A thick barrier-type mucus is produced impeding sperm penetration.
- Ovulation is prevented in about 60 per cent of cycles. The remaining cycles remain unchanged (ovulation occurs) and a proportion of these will have a shortened luteal phase.

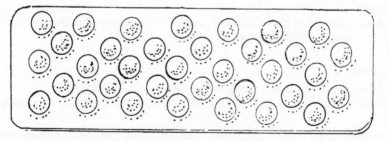

Fig 15.2 Progestogen-only pills – taken every day

Effectiveness
The progestogen-only pill, because of its mode of action, is slightly less effective than the combined pill. With careful use, one woman in 100 will get pregnant in a year. With less careful use, four or more women will get pregnant in a year. The efficacy depends largely on the pill being taken regularly every day of the cycle and at the same time of day.

Advantages
- It can be medically safer than the combined pill as there is no oestrogenic effect.
- It can be used by women over 35 years who smoke.
- It can be used by women with a history of thrombosis.

Disadvantages
- Irregular bleeding – there may be more frequent, prolonged or intermenstrual bleeding or less frequent or missed periods.
- Prolonged amenorrhoea (absence of menstruation) may be experienced by other women. If periods do not return within six months of stopping the pill, medical advice should be sought.
- The pill must be taken regularly. If it is taken more than three hours late, the contraceptive effectiveness is reduced.

Major complications
Should pregnancy occur, the incidence of it being ectopic (outside the uterus, usually in the tube) is increased, but this is still rare.

INJECTABLE HORMONAL CONTRACEPTION
Depo-Provera and Noristerat are long-acting progestogens that are given by deep injection into a muscle during the first five days of the cycle.

Action
It has a similar action to progestogen-only pils.

Effectiveness
Less than one woman in 100 will get pregnant in a year.

Advantages
- Once administered the effect will last for three months (Depo-Provera) and two months (Noristerat).

Disadvantages
- Once the injection has been given, it cannot be removed.
- Side effects may include irregular bleeding, amenorrhoea, or weight gain.
- The return of fertility may be delayed for up to one year or more with Depo-provera.

IMPLANTS

Norplant is a progestogen implant consisting of six small flexible sealed silastic tubes, containing slow release progestogen. The tubes are inserted under the skin in the upper inner aspect of the arm under a local anaesthetic. They are designed to provide contraception for five years.

Effectiveness

Less than 1 woman in 100 will become pregnant in the first year of use. Over the five years about 2 women in 100 will get pregnant.

Side effects

Although the risk of pregnancy is very low, when the method fails there is a slightly increased risk of ectopic pregnancy. Other side effects occur as described for the progestogen-only pill. In addition, there may be local irritation or pain at the site of the implant soon after insertion which then disappears.

Advantages

- The implant offers very effective long-term contraception requiring little user action or attention.
- The advantage over injectable progestogens is that the implant can be removed if severe side effects occur.

Disadvantages

- It requires insertion and removal by a doctor.
- It is an invasive procedure.
- It is costly to the health service and so not always available to women.

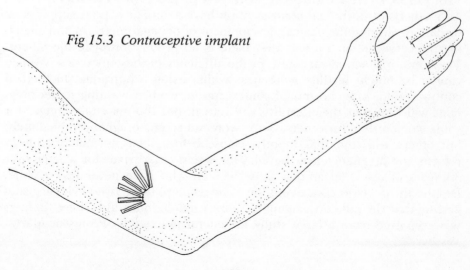

Fig 15.3 Contraceptive implant

INTRA-UTERINE SYSTEM (IUS)

The intra-uterine system is a small plastic device containing progestogen which is inserted through the cervix into the uterus by a doctor. A woman can check it herself by feeling for the threads high in the vagina. The IUS acts mainly by preventing sperm from reaching the ovum. Its secondary action prevents implantation.

Effectiveness

Less than 1 woman in 100 will become pregnant in one year.

Advantages

■ It is effective from the time of insertion.
■ It is designed to prevent pregnancy for at least three years.
■ Periods will be lighter.
■ Unlike the IUD it can be used by women with very heavy painful periods.

Disadvantages

■ There may be temporary side effects such as breast tenderness and acne related to the progestogen.
■ In the first three months erratic light bleeding may occur.

Fertility Awareness in IUS users

Women who have used the progestogen-containing IUD – the IUS – may notice that periods were lighter when the device was in place but on its removal, return to normal. The progestogen component of the device must be considered by women changing to natural methods. Any cyclic disturbance following removal of the IUS is likely to be similar to that observed by women stopping progestogen-only pills. As the device is relatively new, there is as yet no data to support this.

THE EFFECTS OF HORMONAL CONTRACEPTION ON FERTILITY

All methods of hormonal contraception have a similar action, suppressing ovulation, altering the normal development of the endometrium and changing the cervix in such a way that there is no production of fertile mucus. These multiple actions account for the efficiency of these methods. Women cannot be taught fertility awareness whilst using a hormonal method of contraception. After hormonal contraception, women wanting to get pregnant will find that their fertility will return, but this may take longer for some women than for others. Some women become pregnant immediately, but others will find that months elapse before their normal physiology returns and pregnancy is achieved. This is particularly true for women over 30 years of age, and among those women who have never had a child. Despite the delay in conceiving for some women, there is no evidence suggesting that the pill causes long-term irreversible infertility. These findings were reported from a large study in general practice by Professor Martin Vessey.

Note: All women who are using hormonal contraception by whichever route require regular medical check-ups including weight, blood pressure and cervical smears.

THE INTRA-UTERINE DEVICE (IUD)

The intra-uterine contraceptive device is a small plastic device with a coating of thin copper wire, which is inserted through the cervix into the uterus by a doctor. The device is usually inserted towards the end of a period. All devices have a fine filament or threads attached, which protrude from the cervix into the vagina, where they can be checked. Women who have had at least one child are generally more suited to the method than younger women who have not had any children. IUD's are less suitable for women who have a history of pelvic infection including sexually transmitted infections. This applies equally for women who may be exposed to these risks.

Fig 15.4
Intra-uterine devices

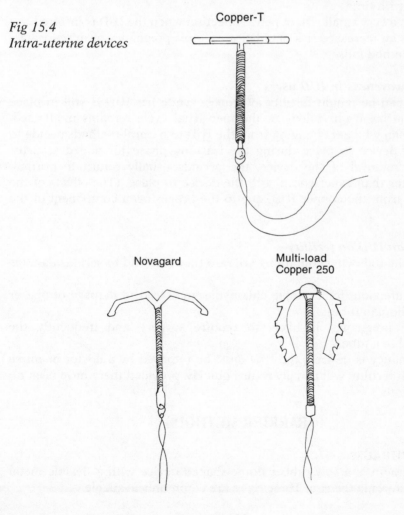

Copper-T

Novagard

Multi-load
Copper 250

Action

The main action of copper IUD's is to prevent sperm from reaching the ovum. The secondary action is to keep the endometrium thin, thus preventing implantation.

Effectiveness

Less than one to two women in 100 will become pregnant in one year.
There is no user failure related to this method.

Advantages

■ The intra-uterine device can remain in place for up to five years or more.
■ It is effective from the time of insertion.

Disadvantages

■ Periods may be heavier, longer and more painful, although this may reduce with time.
■ There is a very small risk of pelvic infection when the IUD is inserted.
■ There is an increased risk of either an ectopic pregnancy or miscarriage if the method fails.

Fertility awareness in IUD users

A woman can be taught fertility awareness while her IUD is still in place because the basic physiology of the menstrual cycle remains unaffected. Some women who are changing from the IUD to natural methods decide to keep their device in place during the learning phase for added security. Following removal of the device, the periods usually return to normal, being lighter than experienced with the device in place. (The effects of the IUS differ from the copper IUD, due to the progestogen component of the device.)

Effects of an IUD on fertility

Although the following conditions are rare they can lead to serious damage to fertility:

■ Pelvic infection, for example chlamydia, may lead to damage of one or both fallopian tubes.
■ Ectopic pregnancy is likely to require surgery and frequently the removal of a tube.

If pregnancy is desired, the IUD must be removed by a doctor or nurse after which fertility will usually return quickly, provided there have been no complications.

BARRIER METHODS

THE DIAPHRAGM

The diaphragm is a soft rubber dome-shaped device with a flexible metal spring reinforcing the rim. Three types are commonly available.

Fig 15.5 The diaphragm

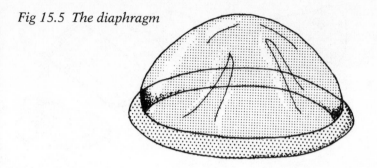

Action

The diaphragm is inserted into the vagina in such a way that the cervix is completely covered. It is held in place by the spring tension of the rim and the vaginal muscles. The front of the diaphragm rests on the pubic bone. When properly positioned, the diaphragm will prevent sperm from reaching the cervix. It should be used with a spermicide. The diaphragm must stay in place for at least six hours after intercourse. It must be fitted initially by a trained doctor or nurse who will give thorough instruction in the use of the method.

Effectiveness

With careful use, four to eight women in 100 will get pregnant in one year. With less careful use, 10–18 women in 100 will get pregnant.

Advantages

- It is medically safe, there is no physiological disturbance to the menstrual cycle.
- It may protect against cancer of the cervix.

Disadvantages

- Some women are sensitive or allergic to the rubber or spermicide.
- Increased incidence of candida or thrush and cystitis.
- Some men complain that they can feel the diaphragm during intercourse.

CERVICAL CAP

A cervical cap may be used in preference to the larger diaphragm. This is useful for women who find diaphragms uncomfortable or who have poor vaginal muscle tone, making the diaphragm unsuitable, or for those women who find cystitis a problem. This may be also be preferred if a male partner complains that a diaphragm can be felt during intercourse. There are three types of cap, depending on the size and shape of the cervix. A cap must be properly fitted by a trained person, when instruction will be given on use of the method. The cervical cap fits snugly over the cervix, held on by suction. Spermicide should be used in conjunction with the cervical cap.

Fig 15.6
The sheath or male condom

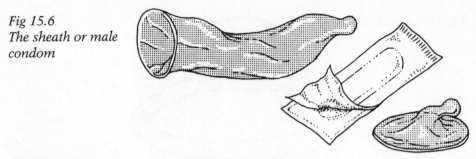

THE CONDOM

The use of condoms is increasing because they provide some protection against sexually transmitted diseases, including HIV (AIDS). The condom is a thin rubber sheath that is put over the erect penis and prevents sperm from entering the woman's vagina.

Effectiveness

Two to 15 women in 100 will get pregnant in one year. The variable use-effectiveness figures generally denote poor technique and inconsistent use.

Rupture of reputable brands of condoms is a rare occurrence. Each country has its own standards of testing. In the UK the BSI kite mark and in Europe the CE mark indicate strict standards of quality control.

Advantages

- The condom allows a man to assume birth control responsibility.
- Condoms are reliable when used properly at every act of intercourse.
- They are easily obtainable from chemists and other stores.
- They give some protection against STD's and may protect against cancer of the cervix.

Disadvantages

- There is an interruption in lovemaking to put on the condom.
- The man must withdraw following ejaculation, before his erection is lost.
- There may be sensitivity or an allergy to the rubber or the spermicide. (Anti-allergic condoms are available.)
- Condoms can only be used for one act of intercourse.
- Oil-based lubricants can damage latex condoms.

THE FEMALE CONDOM

The female condom is a soft, loose, polyurethane sac which lines the vagina. It has an upper ring designed to cover the cervix, rather like a diaphragm, and a lower ring which lies flat against the labia. The material used is stronger than the male condom, so is less likely to break.

Effectiveness

There have been no large scale studies to show this, but research suggests that it should be as effective as the male condom.

Advantages
- It can be put in at any time before intercourse.
- It may protect both partners from sexually transmitted diseases, including HIV.

Disadvantages
- It is expensive to buy.
- It may easily slip out of place.
- A new female condom has to be used for each act of intercourse.

SPERMICIDES

Spermicides are chemical substances which are placed high in the vagina. They act by immobilising sperms, leaving them unlikely to be able to cause fertilisation. Spermicides may be in the form of pessaries, foams, gels or creams. They should only be used in conjunction with a condom or diaphragm.

Some spermicides, like oil-based lubricants and certain medicated pessaries, will damage latex diaphragms and condoms. For this reason, only recommended spermicides should be used.

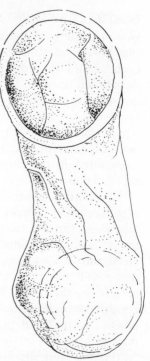

Fig 15.7
The female condom

Advantages
- Spermicides containing Nonoxynol 9 have been shown to inactivate HIV (AIDS virus).
- They are easily available.
- They are relatively free from side effects.

Disadvantages
- Spermicides used alone are unreliable in preventing pregnancy.
- They may cause minor irritations or allergies in either partner.

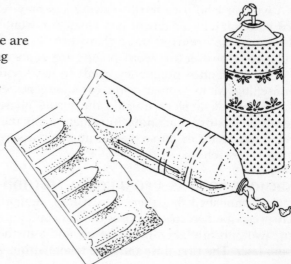

Fig 15.8
Spermicidal creams,
foams and pessaries

FERTILITY AWARENESS AND BARRIER USERS

Is it possible to combine barrier methods with natural methods? It is true that barrier methods certainly do not need to be used on every day of the cycle and a knowledge of fertility awareness will help couples to identify the days when they are fertile. In some family planning clinics it has been recommended that barriers should be used after menstruation, through the pre-ovulatory phase, until the third high temperature is recorded. As the use of spermicides during the pre-ovulatory phase can make the recognition of the mucus symptom difficult, many women use a calendar calculation in combination with the temperature or additionally monitor cervical changes.

Combining barrier use with fertility awareness is often referred to as mixed method use. As women recognise their limits of fertility and time of maximum fertility, many will choose to avoid intercourse completely during the days of fertility maximum. In the 1984 efficiency study, Dr Petra Frank-Hermann in Germany found that among the 851 participants, 506 were using NFP and 245 were mixed method users, who occasionally used barriers during the fertile phase. She observed that many mixed method users continued to have occasional unprotected intercourse during the fertile phase and deduced that the use of barrier methods does not reduce risk-taking.

Barrier methods and spermicides have no adverse effect on the future fertility of a couple.

EMERGENCY CONTRACEPTION

Post-coital contraception is an emergency measure used in cases of unprotected intercourse or contraceptive accident. Depending on the day in the menstrual cycle on which intercourse took place, it will act by preventing fertilisation or implantation.

A woman who uses fertility awareness may realise whether intercourse took place on a fertile day or not. No action would be required if unprotected intercourse occurred more than three days after the calculated day of ovulation. However any woman suffering acute anxiety about the possibility of an unplanned pregnancy needs to have both professional advice and counselling. Many women come for emergency contraception where intercourse has taken place outside the fertile phase. After taking a detailed menstrual history, including information on the regularity and length of cycles, the doctor or nurse may be able to reassure the woman that no pregnancy is possible.

HORMONE PILLS AS A POST-COITAL METHOD

If it is established that there is a risk of unplanned pregnancy, the doctor may prescribe two special doses of pills containing oestrogen and progestogen. Two pills are taken immediately and a further two pills to be taken 12 hours later. The first dose must be taken within 72 hours of a single act of unprotected intercourse. Some women may feel sick after taking these pills because of the high oestrogen content. The nausea may be reduced if the pills are taken with food. Further advice should be sought if vomiting occurs as the tablets will need repeating.

THE INTRA-UTERINE DEVICE AS A POST-COITAL METHOD
A woman may be fitted with a copper IUD within five days of exposure to pregnancy to prevent implantation of the fertilised ovum. This may be suitable for women who are too late to take emergency pills or who dislike or are unable to take hormones. Once fitted, the IUD can be used as a long term contraceptive. IUD's are not suitable for all women.

EFFICIENCY OF EMERGENCY CONTRACEPTION
The failure rate for post-coital pills is up to five per cent.
The IUD is almost 100 per cent effective.

RISK-TAKING
In 'Pandora's Clock' (William Heinemann Ltd, 1993), a book looking at the choices couples face over family planning, there is a wide and puzzling gap between the way people talk about family planning in public and the stories to which they admit in private. In the official version, the couple has no problem with contraception, children are planned and wanted and all decisions are shared. In reality, couples fail to make responsible decisions, take risks and are ambivalent in their emotions and actions. Does this account for the high user failure rates and large number of unplanned pregnancies?

STERILISATION

A couple contemplating sterilisation should understand the implications of the chosen operation. It is the final step, terminating their fertility. A couple should be adequately counselled, usually by their general practitioner, the family planning doctor, or the doctor who is to perform the operation, to ensure that both partners are confident and happy about their decision. It is important for couples to consider the value of fertility in their lives and how loss of fertility may affect self-esteem.

MALE STERILISATION BY VASECTOMY
Vasectomy is a minor operation, usually performed under local anaesthetic, which divides each vas deferens as it passes through the scrotum thus preventing sperm from reaching the exterior. Sperm production continues, but they are absorbed naturally at the blind end of the vas deferens. Sexual intercourse is not physically impaired as fluid from the seminal vesicles and the prostate gland is still ejaculated at orgasm. Additional contraceptive precautions should be taken until two consecutive semen analyses show that there are no remaining sperm in the ejaculate. This may take up to three months or longer.

Vasectomy is an increasingly common means of limiting a family. The incidence of failure is extremely low, but it may occur if the ends of the vas deferens rejoin. Vasectomy fails within a few months of the operation in one in 1,000 cases. This usually shows up in sperm tests. In very rare cases, about one in 3,000 to one in 7,000, vasectomy fails some time later, resulting in unintended pregnancy.

Vasectomy should be considered irreversible, but in practice, reversal of vasectomy may be possible using microsurgical techniques. However, after five or six years, even if the sperm ducts are successfully rejoined, fertility may not always be restored, as in some cases anti-sperm antibodies are produced which destroy the sperm in the testes. There is about a one in three success rate leading to conception.

FEMALE STERILISATION OR TUBAL LIGATION

Female sterilisation is a relatively minor operation, during which the fallopian tubes are closed. This closure will prevent sperm from reaching the ovum at the outer end of the tube, so that conception is not possible. Pregnancy after female sterilisation is very rare, and can only occur if one of the fallopian tubes re-unites. The operation should be considered irreversible. If reversal techniques are attempted at a later date, for example following remarriage, it is most likely to be successful where there has been minimal tubal damage, for example where clips have been used.

NEW FAMILY PLANNING METHODS FOR THE LATE 1990s

Research into family planning continues both in the development of new products and further refinements to existing products. 1996 should see the introduction of safer polyurethane male condoms, new oral contraceptives and a two-rod progestogen implant. An exciting development is in natural family planning with the introduction of the Unipath 'Personal Contraceptive System', a fertility monitor currently on trial. This product, which is discussed further in the section on research, could make a major contribution to family planning.

UNPLANNED PREGNANCIES

Although contraception is widely available, there are more unplanned pregnancies in the UK than in other countries in Western Europe. An unplanned pregnancy is not necessarily unwanted, and may in fact lead to the birth of a much-loved child.

There are three options available with an unplanned pregnancy:
- To continue with the pregnancy and keep the baby.
- To continue with the pregnancy and have the baby adopted.
- To terminate the pregnancy.

TERMINATION OF PREGNANCY
Abortion law of 1967

Laws relating to termination of pregnancy or abortion vary in different countries. In England, the 1967 Abortion Law stated that abortion is allowed up to the 28th week of pregnancy in the following circumstances:

- The continuance of the pregnancy would involve risk to the life of the pregnant woman greater than if the pregnancy were terminated.
- The continuance of the pregnancy would involve risk of injury to the physical or mental health of the pregnant woman greater than if the pregnancy were terminated.
- The continuance of the pregnancy would involve risk of injury to the physical or mental health of the existing child(ren) of the family of the pregnant woman greater than if the pregnancy were terminated.
- There is substantial risk that if the child were born it would suffer from such physical or mental abnormalities as to be seriously handicapped.

The Human Fertilisation and Embryology Act of 1990

The 1967 Abortion Law was amended in 1990 in the Human Fertilisation and Embryology Act which reduced the time limit for abortion to the 24th week of pregnancy in most circumstances. However it permitted abortion without time limits in the following categories:

- To prevent grave permanent injury to the physical or mental health of the pregnant woman.
- When there is risk to the life of the pregnant woman greater than if the pregnancy were terminated.
- Where there is a substantial risk that if the child were born it would suffer from such physical or mental abnormalities as to be seriously handicapped.

BETH AND JERRY: Beth rang the NFP teacher for an appointment. She wanted to learn about fertility because she desperately wanted a baby. She found it difficult to talk about what had happened two years ago, without bursting into tears. Both she and Jerry had been so happy when she became pregnant and then came the worry of contact with German measles, a blood test, and the advice to terminate the pregnancy. Jerry had been a great support. 'It's the only thing we can do,' he tried to comfort her. 'We will have another baby right away.' But now it was nearly two years later and she wasn't pregnant. Beth started charting, and was reassured by the temperature shift and good mucus symptoms. At the third interview she was more relaxed. She now wanted to talk about the abortion. There were many questions to be answered about the operation, and many fears to be expressed, among others that she might be infertile, and would never have another child. Beth conceived three months later and after a normal pregnancy she and Jerry were delighted with the birth of a daughter.

Counselling should always be offered before an abortion is performed, to discuss the woman's/couple's feelings about the pregnancy, and the effect that the abortion may have, in both the short and long term.

Procedures for termination of pregnancy
Medical method
■ Up to 63 days from a woman's last menstrual period (LMP), mifepristone, a potent anti-progesterone compound, can be used in combination with a vaginal prostaglandin, for the medical termination of pregnancy. There will be some abdominal pain for several hours and vaginal bleeding comparable to a heavy period.

Surgical method
■ Between seven and 12 weeks of pregnancy, the procedure normally involves a general anaesthetic, and dilatation of the cervix followed by either suction aspiration or curettage, to remove the fetus and placenta.
■ Between 12 and 16 weeks, the surgical method involves dilatation and curettage (D & C).
■ After 16 weeks of pregnancy, abortion is induced by various means and the foetus will be expelled, after several hours of uterine contractions, in a recognisable state.

A single abortion carried out under ideal medical conditions should not cause any short- or long-term physical effects. Complications of repeat abortions include infection which may spread to the fallopian tubes, affecting future fertility, and damage to the cervix resulting in an incompetent cervix and subsequent repeated miscarriages. Perforation of the uterus, although very rare, is a major complication.

Psychological adjustment to abortion depends largely on the personal circumstances, and the level of support from family or friends. Abortion in the first eight weeks generally results in less psychological trauma and regret than later abortions. Post-abortion counselling should always be available.

16. Vaginal Infections, Sexually Transmitted Diseases and Cancer

Information about sexually transmitted diseases (STDs) is included in this book, because fertility is so easily damaged by these infections. It is important that everyone should understand these health hazards and be prepared to pass on their information to others.

Sexually transmitted disease refers to any infection that is acquired during sexual contact or intercourse. Education in fertility awareness can make it easier to understand how STDs may damage future fertility.

Throughout the world, the spread of STDs has been one of the major disappointments in public health in the last two decades. World-wide, 365,000 people become infected each day. In the UK, 700,000 people become infected each year.

Symptoms may be very slight or absent in women, especially in the early stages of infection. Frequently the first symptom is a vaginal discharge. Observations of cervical mucus will be masked by the infected discharge, resulting in difficulty in interpreting the mucus pattern. If the infection spreads to involve the cervix, causing cervicitis (inflammation of the cervix), then the cervical mucus will also be affected.

A woman who has learnt fertility awareness will be quickly alerted to any change which may indicate infection, and she will be in a position to seek prompt medical aid. Treatment in special clinics is completely confidential. If medication is indicated, the course of treatment should be completed as directed, even though symptoms may have been relieved. Abstinence should be observed for the duration of the symptoms and for the time of treatment, as intercourse may cause the infection to spread to neighbouring organs, such as the urinary system. The sexual partner may also be infected

No one is immune to STDs, and re-infection can occur as soon as the treatment ends. With early diagnosis and appropriate treatment, most sexually transmitted diseases are completely curable.

CANDIDIASIS OR VAGINAL THRUSH

Most women will experience an attack of thrush (fungal or yeast infection of the vagina) at some stage in their lives. It may be acquired sexually, but also frequently occurs without sexual transmission. Any condition which alters the normally acid environment of the vagina may predispose to thrush, including:

■ Antibiotics – the normal lacto-bacillae present in the vagina may be destroyed.
■ Certain diets.

- Pregnancy.
- Diabetes.
- Tight jeans, nylon tights and pants as these increase perspiration.
- Vaginal irritants, for example perfumed soaps, bubble baths and vaginal deodorants.

Symptoms include an intense itching of the vulva or vagina, with or without a thick white curdy discharge. Small white curds may be seen on the vaginal walls, and there may be soreness and pain on passing urine. Treatment is usually given in the form of antifungal pessaries, for example clotrimazole (Canesten) pessaries placed high in the vagina as directed, plus Canesten cream for the vulval skin. The male partner should also apply the cream to his penis. Some women may have troublesome recurrent episodes of thrush requiring further investigation.

TRICHOMONIASIS

This is a parasitic organism which infects the ridged vaginal lining, causing an intense itching just inside the reddened vagina and a profuse, frothy greenish-yellow offensive discharge. The usual treatment is a course of oral metronidazole (Flagyl) tablets for both partners.

NON-SPECIFIC URETHRITIS (NSU)

Non-specific urethritis is a term used to describe inflammation of the urethra of unknown origin, although chlamydia is a frequent cause. It affects both men and women. It may arise by chance or be sexually transmitted.

Symptoms may include frequent, painful urination, often within 24 hours of intercourse taking place, pain during intercourse and possibly a white or yellowish vaginal discharge. If the infection is mild, a woman may be symptom-free. Treatment includes antibiotics for both partners if necessary.

CHLAMYDIA INFECTIONS

Chlamydia infections are becoming increasingly common. Chlamydia bacteria are known to be responsible for a number of infections, many of which are not transmitted sexually. Among the sexually transmitted diseases affecting the male are non-specific urethritis and lympho-granuloma venereum, a disease causing swelling of the lymph glands in the groin. Chlamydia can affect male fertility.

In the female, if the infection is not treated, it may travel up the reproductive tract causing cervicitis, and salpingitis. This pathogen is responsible for 70 per cent of pelvic inflammatory disease (PID), which can result in tubal infertility. PID is also responsible for a high proportion of ectopic pregnancies. Treatment involves a course of antibiotics such as tetracycline.

GENITAL HERPES

Genital herpes is caused by herpes simplex virus type 2. (Type 1 usually causes the common coldsore of the mouth or nose.) Genital herpes occurs either as an isolated attack or more commonly as a recurring infection. The first attack, which usually occurs 2–12 days after sexual intercourse with an infected person, is generally the most serious, lasting for two to three weeks. Recurrent attacks are usually milder, lasting 5–10 days. Symptoms include an itching or burning sensation of the genitals, followed two days later by multiple blisters of the vulva, vagina, cervix or rectum. These painful blisters burst in around three days, forming small ulcers with a crust, which heal within two to three weeks.

An attack may be brought on by stress, or being 'run down' in some individuals. There may be a general feeling of ill health, with flu-like symptoms, headache, backache, pains down the thighs and a raised temperature accompanying the blisters. Genital contact and intercourse should be avoided while the tingling sensation and blisters last, to prevent transmission of the virus. There is no specific cure for genital herpes at present, although treatment with acyclovir (Zovirax) will alleviate the symptoms of an attack.

GENITAL WARTS

Genital warts are multiple small growths of skin on the vulva and possibly around the anus, or on the cervix. They are usually, but not always, acquired sexually due to entry of the wart virus through small fissures in the skin or mucus membrane. Symptoms will not be apparent for between two weeks and eight months after the virus was contracted.

Effective treatment includes application of podophyllin paint to the warts. Special care is needed during pregnancy, as genital warts can spread rapidly.

GONORRHOEA

Gonorrhoea is caused by transmission of the gonococcus bacterium during sexual activity. As with most sexually transmitted diseases, because of anatomical differences the male partner is more likely to show symptoms of the disease.

A woman frequently has no symptoms, unless there is an accompanying infection, for example trichomoniasis, in which case the symptoms of this infection will predominate. A woman may have gonorrhoea and unknowingly infect her sexual partner(s). If symptoms are present, they include frequent painful urination and a discharge from the urethra 5–10 days after the infection was contracted. Treatment usually involves a single injection of a slow release penicillin. If the organism is resistant to penicillin, oral tetracycline may be given.

SYPHILIS

The incidence of syphilis is now very low. It is caused by a spiral-shaped bacterium which leads to the formation of sores or chancres. The sores usually appear at the site of contact. Women are frequently unaware of the hardened, red-rimmed, painless sores, which will disappear within a few weeks even without treatment. If this stage of the disease is untreated, infection of the blood will follow within a few months. The second stage of the disease, which lasts from three to six months, will produce symptoms of skin rashes, enlarged lymph glands, fever, sore throat, headaches and many other symptoms associated with generalised infection of the blood and body organs. If the infection remains untreated at this stage, between 10–20 years later tertiary syphilis will develop, resulting in damage to the heart, brain, spinal cord and eyes, causing blindness.

Treatment of syphilis is with penicillin or tetracycline. If it is treated in the primary or secondary stages, permanent damage will be prevented.

All pregnant women are routinely screened for syphilis and gonorrhoea in antenatal clinics, because of the very severe consequences for the developing foetus infected with these diseases.

AIDS (Acquired Immune Deficiency Syndrome)

HISTORY
AIDS was first described in the United States in 1981. At first it was associated with male homosexuality, but it is now predominantly a heterosexual disorder.

PREVALENCE
It is devastating Africa and is spreading rapidly in the United States, and to a lesser extent in Europe. It is impossible to assess the prevalence of HIV in the UK, because the policy of confidentiality precludes the collecting of accurate statistics. However, the number of people suffering from fully developed AIDS is, so far, less than the number projected.

VIRUS
It is caused by HIV or human immuno-deficiency virus. The virus enters the T cells. These are lymphocytes, white blood cells, which carry suitable receptors to attract the virus. These T cells are part of the body's immune defence system to combat infection. Once in the cell, the virus reproduces itself and penetrates the DNA, where it becomes a permanent part of the cell nucleus. The virus remains dormant for a variable time, and there is no known way of eradicating it.

TRANSMISSION
HIV can only be transmitted by sexual intercourse or by direct injection into the body. Haemophiliacs have been infected by blood transfusions or

injections with Factor VIII, a blood product. Drug users can be infected by sharing needles. Very rarely health workers have been infected by accidental needle stab. It cannot be caught by kissing, or by using crockery or cutlery that has been used by an infected person. It is not caught from toilet seats and it is not spread by ordinary activities in school or at work.

AIDS AND PREGNANCY

Mothers infected by HIV can transmit the infection to the baby during pregnancy. The virus can also be transmitted in breast milk.

COURSE OF HIV INFECTION

People infected by HIV react in different ways. Some have a brief illness, similar to influenza or glandular fever, between four weeks and four months from the time of infection. After that many people remain symptom-free for many years and some may never develop AIDS, but the majority become ill between three and 10 years from the time that they were infected. People do not die of AIDS itself, but of AIDS related illnesses such as:

■ Candidiasis of the oesophagus or lungs.
■ Cytomegalo-virus infection, which becomes widespread throughout the body.
■ Herpes simplex spreading to the oesophagus.
■ Cerebral lymphoma or encephalitis.
■ Kaposi's sarcoma – a skin cancer.
■ Tuberculosis.

Symptoms include profound fatigue, weight-loss, fever, night sweats, swollen glands and skin rashes.

TREATMENT

People who are HIV positive require support from their relatives, friends and those around them and they should be encouraged to lead normal lives. Treatment should be given immediately to alleviate any symptoms as they arise and so prevent debilitation.

RESEARCH

There are massive programmes of research in many countries to find new drugs to treat those who have been infected with HIV, and also to find a vaccine which will protect people against this terrible disease.

There have been a number of reports concerning people who have been exposed to HIV but have not become infected. It has been discovered that a very small number of the at-risk population are immune to the virus. Dr Sarah Rowland Jones is carrying out research in Africa amongst a number of prostitutes who have been highly exposed to HIV, but have not contracted the infection. She is hoping to discover the factors responsible for their immunity which could lead to the development of a vaccine.

HIV TESTING

Those who have been exposed to the possibility of infection with the virus should be offered HIV testing at once and again three months after exposure. The tests should also be offered to their sexual partners. They should be encouraged to have the tests, because in spite of the hardships experienced by those who discover they are infected, there is still much that can be done.

CONCLUSION

AIDS and HIV infection are not notifiable diseases. In this country there are thousands of men and women who are HIV positive. Most of them are unaware that they have the virus and can transmit it to others. Therein lies the danger. The AIDS epidemic can only be contained if people understand the value of forming stable relationships and act responsibly to protect themselves and others.

HEPATITIS B

Hepatitis B is transmitted in a similar way to HIV. It causes infection of the liver. A vaccine is available against hepatitis B for high-risk groups and gives protection for at least five years.

TO SUMMARISE

Education in fertility awareness can help men and women to understand the importance of protecting themselves from sexually transmitted diseases. This education will also help them to understand the possible effects of these diseases on their future fertility. Any individual who has unusual symptoms, or who thinks he or she may have contracted a sexually transmitted disease, should see a doctor promptly, or contact the nearest special clinic.

Signs and symptoms related to sexual infection include the following:
- Discharge from the penis.
- Any unusual vaginal discharge.
- Frequent or painful urination.
- Pain in the lower abdomen – any severe pain, especially if it becomes worse after intercourse, may indicate pelvic infection (pelvic inflammatory disease).
- Unexplained sores, ulcers, or warts in the mouth, or on the genitals.

It should be emphasised that there may be other explanations for the symptoms apart from sexual infection – for example, urinary symptoms may be caused by cystitis, which is very common in women – but medical advice is always necessary for accurate diagnosis and effective treatment.

CANCER

CANCER OF THE CERVIX

The number of women suffering from cancer of the cervix is increasing. There are certain known risk factors including:

■ Many sexual partners.
■ More than five years on the contraceptive pill.
■ Sexually transmitted diseases.
■ Smoking

Certain strains of wart virus, or Human Papilloma Virus, HPV, are thought to cause pre-cancerous changes in cervical cells which are evident on a cervical smear. It takes between five and 10 years from the first appearance of changes in cervical cytology to the development of invasive cancer if the condition is untreated.

If early pre-cancerous cells are detected by cervical smear, a repeat smear will usually be taken, followed by a colposcopy. This is a procedure used to examine the vagina and cervix under magnification through an instrument known as a colposcope. Appropriate treatment will be given according to the findings. This may involve destruction of the affected tissue by cryosurgery (freezing) or laser therapy. If the abnormal cells seem more extensive, a cone biopsy may be performed to remove damaged cells from the cervix and to determine the extent of the invasion. In advanced cases, hysterectomy may be the only effective method of treatment.

ENDOMETRIAL CANCER

There is an increased risk of endometrial cancer (cancer of the uterine lining) in older women, although this is much less common than cervical cancer. Heavy prolonged bleeding with clots in pre-menopausal cycles or bleeding in post-menopausal women should always be investigated.

17. Scientific Research and New Technologies

THE CHANCES OF CONCEPTION THROUGHOUT THE MENSTRUAL CYCLE

USING THE DAY OF TEMPERATURE SHIFT AS A MARKER OF OVULATION

In the late 1960s a study was conducted by Professor John Marshall and Dr John Barrett to analyse the chances of conception following intercourse on different days of the menstrual cycle. A total of 241 married couples who had proved their fertility by the birth of at least one child participated in the study. The women's ages ranged from 20–49 years. Some of the couples were using their knowledge of fertility to avoid pregnancy, others to conceive, and still others changed their intentions during the course of the study, from avoiding to planning a further pregnancy.

The women were asked to record their temperature each morning and to record each act of intercourse on their charts. All the data from the charts were computerised. As each couple might have intercourse on several different days in a particular cycle, subsequent conception could not immediately be attributed to a single act of intercourse, therefore a very complex mathematical analysis was involved to produce the results.

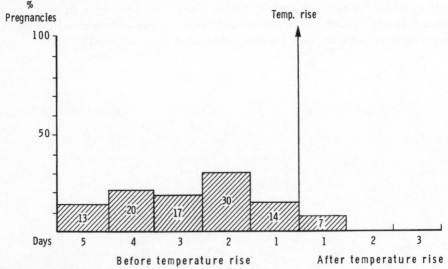

Fig 17.1 Chances of conception in relation to the temperature rise
(Marshall & Barrett 1969)

It should be noted that in this study, for convenience only, the days were counted before and after the temperature shift, realising that ovulation could not be pinpointed with accuracy.

The results showed that the risks of conception were effectively limited to the five days before the temperature rise and the first day of an elevated temperature. The chance of conception occurring outside these limits approximated to zero.

This study confirmed the impression that the chances of conception following intercourse after the temperature rise are much lower than before the rise. The chance of conception is at its greatest several days prior to the temperature rise, hence the significantly higher user failure rate associated with intercourse in the pre-ovulatory phase.

Using these statistics, a calculation was made to determine the effect of the frequency of intercourse on the chances of conception. If couples are unaware of, or disregard the cyclic phases of fertility and infertility and intercourse takes place at random, the chances of conception will be directly proportional to the frequency of intercourse. Couples who have intercourse once per week have a 14 per cent chance of conceiving in any particular cycle. The chance of conception increases to a maximum of 68 per cent for couples who have intercourse every day.

The results of the Marshall and Barrett study provide valuable supportive evidence when explaining the pregnancy risks to couples or when discussing the chances of pregnancy with subfertile couples.

USING HORMONAL ASSAYS
In 1994 a similar study was carried out by Weinberg and Wilcox. They used hormonal assays on daily urine samples to estimate the time of ovulation. They showed that it was possible for conception to occur from the sixth day before ovulation and on the day of ovulation itself. The chances of conception fell to zero 24 hours after ovulation.

CERVICAL MUCUS

Research in the field of infertility in particular has confirmed that if sperm are to penetrate cervical mucus to achieve conception, the mucus must possess certain characteristics.

In 1964 Chretien examined cervical mucus on each day of a woman's menstrual cycle, and using the electron microscope showed that it is composed of filaments of different diameter – thin, medium and thick.

Following menstruation, during the early relatively infertile phase, when the mucus is thick and sticky and forming a plug in the cervical canal, it is seen to be composed of filaments of medium diameter forming a dense network.

During the fertile phase as the volume of mucus increases under the influence of oestrogen, becoming thinner, clear and stretchy (the 'Spinnbarkeit effect'), it is seen to be composed of all three types of filament stretched out

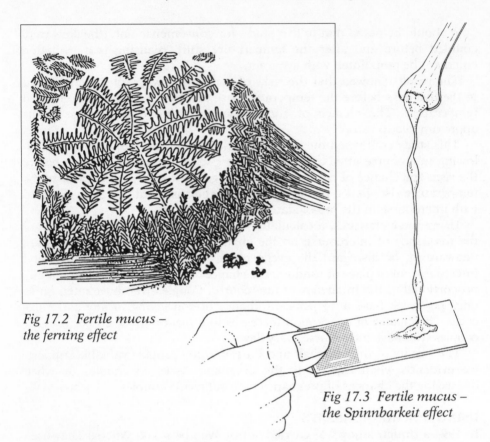

*Fig 17.2 Fertile mucus –
the ferning effect*

*Fig 17.3 Fertile mucus –
the Spinnbarkeit effect*

to form a very loose network. This mucus is easily penetrated by sperm.

During the post-ovulatory infertile phase, under the influence of progesterone, the mucus thickens and forms an even denser plug, blocking the
cervical canal. This mucus is also composed of all three types of filament,
but these are tightly woven together, forming an impenetrable barrier to
sperm.

Observation of the structure of mucus in the cervical canal requires specialised techniques and skills. Inevitably the characteristics of cervical
mucus, when it appears at the vulva, will have undergone changes due to
the drying effect of the lower vagina and the time taken for the secretions to
pass along the ridged vaginal lining. Samples of mucus taken from the cervical os crystallise as they are dried on a glass slide. Under a microscope the
'ferning pattern', which is characteristic of fertile mucus, is seen.

Professor Odeblad, who has been investigating cervical mucus since the
late 1950s, has made a major contribution to the practical understanding of
the complex properties of cervical mucus. He has developed a biophysical
hypothesis, concerned with the way in which sperm travel through the cervical mucus in ascending the female reproductive tract, so that fertilisation
can take place. He postulates that fertile mucus facilitates the passage of
actively motile sperm, and filters out those that are defective or damaged.

USE OF ULTRASOUND SCANS AND HORMONE ASSAYS TO DETECT THE FERTILE PHASE

A study was made in 1984 by Dr Anna Flynn in Birmingham to compare a woman's subjective assessment of the fertile period (by sympto-thermal charting) with urinary hormone levels and detection of ovulation by ultrasound.

The study participants were eight healthy fertile women aged from 25–35 years, who were experienced users of the sympto-thermal method. All the women were asked to observe and record changes in the temperature, mucus and cervix and to note ovulation pain or breast tenderness. Each woman deduced her probable fertile time from these sympto-thermal indicators. Measurements of the hormones oestrogen, progesterone, follicle stimulating hormone (FSH) and luteinising hormone (LH) were made using daily specimens of early morning urine. Ultrasound scans were begun on the day of the cycle the women estimated to be the beginning of their fertile phase, as defined by the first appearance of mucus or S minus 20, whichever came first. Daily scans were performed to determine the number and size of follicles and to observe ovulation.

When ultrasound waves are directed towards the ovaries, an image of the fluid-filled follicle can be observed. The immature follicle, (only a few millimetres in size) grows to reach full maturity, (about 2cm). The ovum is released and the follicle collapses to form the corpus luteum. Ovulation day was considered to be the day after maximum follicular growth was observed.

The study concluded that the most reliable clinical indicator to detect the beginning of the fertile phase was the calendar calculation S minus 20. Mucus was not always present sufficiently early to warn of approaching fertility, if the couple wished to avoid conception. One pregnancy resulted from intercourse on a dry day (calculated by ultrasound and hormone assays to be five days before ovulation). It was reasonably assumed that if the S minus 20 rule had been applied, the pregnancy might not have occurred as intercourse would have been discontinued two days previously. The double check of the first appearance of mucus or S minus 20, whichever comes first, appeared to offer the most reliable combination of indicators. Hormone assays (measurements) did not increase the reliability of detecting the beginning of the fertile phase.

In this study the end of the fertile phase was identified as the morning of the third high temperature or evening of the fourth day after the peak mucus symptom, whichever came last. In a very small number of cycles one or other of the indicators (mucus or temperature) fell within the fertile limits defined by hormone assays or ultrasound, but it was considered that using the double check methodology, very few unplanned pregnancies would be expected. This study highlighted the accuracy of a woman's subjective assessment of the fertile phase and reconfirmed scientifically the validity of the sympto-thermal guidelines.

In 1986 another small study carried out in Cardiff by Dr Robert Ryder, Colleen Norman and others was conducted along similar lines to the Birmingham study. Six women of proven fertility who were NFP users recorded a total of 15 menstrual cycles on sympto-thermal charts. Their subjective assessment of their fertility was compared with measurements of luteinising hormone levels and the time of ovulation was estimated on ultrasound scan, assuming the day of ovulation as the day before the appearance of the corpus luteum. Three cycles out of the 15 were suggestive of persistent luteinised unruptured follicles (LUF).

The researchers commented that the most accurate means of pinpointing ovulation was by identifying the day of the most abundant fertile-type mucus. This was as accurate as LH measurements. This finding could be most helpful for couples with fertility problems who wish to maximise their chances of conception.

The day before the temperature shift coincided with the day of ovulation in eight out of 12 cycles. This was further confirmation of the accuracy of the sympto-thermal guidelines for detecting the onset of the post-ovulatory infertile phase. The study suggested that when natural family planning methods fail it is not due to the unreliability of the method, but to user failure.

SEX DETERMINATION

The sex of a child is determined by the father at the time of conception, when either an X chromosome or a Y chromosome sperm fertilises the ovum to produce a girl or a boy respectively.

According to the work of Dr Shettles, an American gynaecologist, the timing of intercourse in relation to the quality of cervical mucus is a crucial factor in sex determination. Around the time of ovulation, the alkaline peak mucus provides the optimum conditions for sperm survival of both types of sperm. The Y sperm are lighter than the X sperm, and able to move more rapidly towards the ovum, so the chances of a boy are increased by a single act of intercourse on peak day or the day following peak, as close as possible to the predicted ovulation.

A single act of intercourse two to three days before ovulation, when fertile mucus signs are just beginning, at the transition from thick, cloudy mucus to thin, transparent mucus increases the chances of a girl. The less alkaline medium of early transition mucus favours the survival of the more acid-resistant X chromosome sperms.

Two further studies confirming the work of Shettles were carried out by Dr Leonie McSweeney in Nigeria, where the preference for the eldest child to be a male puts unbearable pressures on the wives.

Other studies, however, have not supported this theory. At least 30 other variables that may influence sex have been reported, such as the rising female birth-rate with increasing parental age. It is also suggested that there is an increasing male birth-rate with higher socio-economic status, and frequency of intercourse. Books and magazine articles about the timing of intercourse and the effect of acid or alkaline douching have brought the subject of sex determination to the public eye. Couples have nothing to lose by testing out this theory, but they should be aware of the realistic chances. The percentage change in sex ratio achieved by these measures is probably only altered by around 5–10 per cent, and 50 per cent of the couples will achieve the sex of their choice anyway.

DIAGNOSTIC TESTS TO PREDICT THE FERTILE PHASE OF THE CYCLE

There has been a lot of research on the development of simple urinary assays to determine the limits of the fertile phase. The changing oestrogen/progesterone ratio is proving difficult to refine to a simple yet effective test.

The Progesturine TM PDG identifies the onset of the post-ovulatory infertile phase. It is not yet simplified for use in the home, but could be a substitute for temperature recordings. There is not, as yet, any technological means of determining the onset of the fertile phase in the form of a home kit.

THE OVARIAN MONITOR
Professor James Brown, who works with Drs John and Evelyn Billings in Australia, has developed the ovarian monitor. This measures daily urinary oestrogen and pregnanediol levels in order to identify the periods of fertility and infertility during the menstrual cycle. Testing has been satisfactory and it is hoped that home kits will be made available.

THE PERSONAL CONTRACEPTIVE SYSTEM
A birth control monitor has been developed by scientists working for Unipath and is possibly the most important advance in the field of natural family planning. It is based on dipstick immuno-assay technology which Unipath have already applied in their products 'Clearplan' – for the detection of the LH surge – and 'Clearblue' – the pregnancy test. The dipstick carries reagents that simultaneously measure the levels of urinary oestrogens and LH.

The hand-held monitor has a display panel which shows a green light during the infertile phase, or a red light during the fertile phase. Clinical trials are continuing and it is hoped that this device will be available for women to use in their own homes shortly. The developers claim that no special training is required to use this system and for most women only eight days per cycle need to be tested.

TECHNOLOGICAL DEVICES BASED ON THERMAL CHANGES DURING THE CYCLE

The Rite-time rhythm clock is a computerised electronic thermometer. The daily temperature is measured by a sensitive probe and the reading is displayed on a screen. The data is stored in the computer and is used to indicate the beginning of the post-ovulatory infertile phase. It does not predict the onset of the fertile phase. Clinical trials in the UK have shown the Rite-time to be reliable.

The Bioself Fertility Indicator is a similar device to the Rite-time, but it uses a combination of a calendar calculation and temperature readings to define the limits of the fertile phase. The temperature readings are not displayed but instead the fertile and infertile phases of the cycle are indicated by means of a red or green light. This device was tested in the UK by Dr Anna Flynn and her colleagues and was found to be reliable.

Evidence suggests that the blood flow to the hands is reduced prior to ovulation, lowering the temperature and closing off the smaller blood vessels. A device which monitors the blood flow is being developed.

SALIVA AND MUCUS TESTING

Other research projects have investigated means of assessing hormone levels in the saliva and in cervical mucus, in an effort to provide a simple, reliable test for domestic use, that will consistently and accurately predict ovulation and the limits of the fertile phase. Although some products are appearing on the market, they have not been subjected to clinical trials and therefore the reliability is not proven.

POSSIBILITY OF BIRTH DEFECTS

It is periodically suggested that there may be an increased risk of birth defects and miscarriages in NFP users because a high proportion of unplanned pregnancies will result from intercourse at the outer limits of fertility when the sperm or the ovum are aged. The evidence to support this theory was originally from results of animal experiments using aged sperm and ova. At present, there is no definite evidence to suggest an increased incidence of either birth defects or miscarriages in humans in these circumstances.

In a large WHO multicentre trial of the ovulation method, researchers looked at the outcome of 160 pregnancies. They found that the spontaneous abortion rate was 10 per cent lower than the 25 per cent for the general population and the rate of congenital malformation was 1.25 per cent, the same as that for the general population. The study concluded that spontaneous abortions (miscarriages) and congenital malformations or birth defects were not related to the time-interval between sexual intercourse and ovulation.

Couples practising natural family planning have the advantage that the method does not involve the introduction of drugs, chemicals or irritants into the body, so a naturally occurring pregnancy will not be affected by any of these potential hazards.

18. Teaching Fertility Awareness and Natural Family Planning

THE NATURAL FAMILY PLANNING TEACHER

Natural family planning is taught by doctors and nurses and by lay people who have attended a teacher training course held by one of the NFP organisations. Lay teachers require medical support and all teachers require in-service training in order to update their knowledge and skills. The teacher is generally referred to as 'she' in this chapter because most teachers are women. There are a few male teachers and many others who work as part of husband and wife teams.

A teacher needs to be caring and interested in her clients. She must be able to communicate effectively and to understand the importance of confidentiality. She should respect the unique characteristics of her clients and develop a sensitivity to their feelings. She should not try to impose her own views, moral beliefs or values, but using the skills of a good listener she will identify her clients' needs and so be able to support them. A natural family planning teacher should recognise her limitations. She should be quick to identify those problems which are outside her expertise and be prepared to refer clients for medical advice when necessary.

The teacher should be sensitive to the very intimate nature of her work and the observations required. Some women or couples may find difficulty particularly at first in discussing this very private part of their lives. A teacher should see her clients in a comfortable room which affords privacy and is accessible and acceptable to her clients.

TEACHING FERTILITY AWARENESS AND NFP

Teaching is usually given on a one to one or couple to couple basis, but as more people are looking for instruction in fertility awareness and natural methods, programmes for group teaching are increasingly available either through health service outlets or as part of adult education courses. Some couples may feel intimidated by group teaching and find difficulty expressing problems of a sexual nature. It is most important that where education about fertility awareness is given in a group setting, clients also have access to the teacher on an individual basis to ensure their needs are met.

Education in fertility awareness is about giving the client the knowledge, the skills and the confidence to help them to manage their own fertility and family planning. All the factual information necessary for teaching the sympto-thermal method of natural family planning is included in this book. Efficiency depends on the experience and skill of the teacher as much as on the motivation of the client.

TEACHING PROGRAMME

FIRST SESSION

Ideally both partners should be seen together, particularly at the first session to encourage joint responsibility. However, frequently only the woman is seen. The teacher should welcome the client, introducing herself, and her work, and aiming to put her client at ease.

Client history

A careful history should be taken. This will depend largely on the circumstances in which teaching is being given, for example general practice, family planning clinics or by private arrangement. The history should include:

- **Obstetric history** – to establish the number of pregnancies and their outcome, including information about miscarriages or terminations.
- **Menstrual history** – to establish age of menarche, normal menstrual pattern and any problems.
- **Gynaecological history** – to indicate any problems, past or present which may affect fertility, and any gynaecological investigations, including cervical smears, ensuring these are up-to-date.
- **Contraceptive history** – to determine past and present methods of family planning, any problems or personal preferences and the suitability for using a natural method.
- **Medical history** – to include past or current use of medication.
- **Rubella status** – all women should be immune to rubella before they plan pregnancy.

The history taking is important to establish a rapport with the client, ensuring that the teacher understands the needs of her client. It should be done in an informal manner, allowing the client time and space to disclose her history and to explore her family planning needs and intentions.

Family planning intention

While some clients will be clear about their intention to achieve or to avoid a pregnancy or how they wish to use their increased knowledge about fertility, others will have very ambivalent feelings – some expressed and others unexpressed. Many clients who stop contraception and change to natural methods are doing so at a time when they would like to start a family in the near future. The definition of 'near' frequently varies between partners. Discrepancies in motives should be explored with great sensitivity.

Efficiency

Couples wishing to avoid pregnancy should understand that, like other methods, NFP is not guaranteed 100 per cent effective. The efficiency of the method and the factors which influence this can be discussed. A record should be made in the client notes that this has been discussed and understood by the client.

Current knowledge

Before beginning the initial teaching it is very helpful to assess the client's current level of knowledge about her fertility. Many couples have a very patchy understanding of the reproductive process, frequently recalled from school days and rather inadequate or inappropriate sex education. However with increasing interest and literature available on this subject, other couples will have gleaned information from other sources – some reliable and some very questionable! It is useful to elicit the information source and its reliability. Teaching has to be tailored to suit the requirements of the couple and given in accordance with the clients' learning capacity. Lack of education is no barrier to learning the method.

Attitudes

It is important that as part of training courses, teachers are encouraged to consider their own feelings, views and values about NFP and abstinence. In understanding her own perspective, she is then in a better position to understand her clients' viewpoint. It is worth considering the following:

■ Is there a strong religious or moral factor motivating this couple?
■ Do both partners share these views?
■ Are there conflicting interests in using a natural method?

Introducing the client to the basic concepts of fertility awareness

Fertility awareness is important as part of health education at all stages of reproductive life. Many women will benefit greatly from this knowledge, gaining insight and understanding into how cycles can vary at different stages of life and due to outside influences such as stress. All women who receive a basic education in fertility awareness should understand that if they want to put their knowledge to practical use, as a family planning method, they will need to have a full course of instruction.

Anatomy and physiology of the male and female reproductive systems

A very basic understanding of the fundamentals of reproduction is necessary to understand combined fertility and appropriate guidelines for effective family planning. This, as with other teaching, should be adapted to the clients' level of understanding.

Recording the temperature

Women are taught how to record and chart accurate waking temperatures, including use of a fertility or digital thermometer, the route, the time taken and disturbances likely to affect the recordings. Thorough instruction will generally ensure a woman produces accurate temperature readings from the first cycle. Mercury fertility thermometers can be prescribed free of charge on the National Health Service but digital thermometers have to be paid for. Charts can be supplied by the NFP teacher or directly from the NFP service, (see Addresses, page 172).

Observing and charting the mucus symptom

Women should be taught to record the mucus symptom, considering the sensation, the appearance and the colour of her secretions, and recording this on her chart using her own descriptive words. It may take several cycles for a woman to observe this very subjective symptom with confidence. It is important at this stage that the emphasis is on observing the fertility symptoms. The interpretation of these observations is taught at later sessions.

A handout should be given in the form of a book or printed sheet to reinforce the verbal message, so that the client always has clear written instructions available.

Follow-up appointments should be made as appropriate. To help with chart interpretation they should be arranged at approximately monthly intervals, to fit in with the client's cycle where possible. Clients should understand the appointment system and arrangements for further telephone support between sessions if this is needed.

SECOND AND SUBSEQUENT SESSIONS

Chart review

The chart can be interpreted by the teacher at first, but the whole emphasis should be placed on helping the client towards independence in her use of the method. The teacher can use colour as part of chart interpretation to highlight the fertile and infertile phases of the cycle. Many couples find this very visual feature helpful. Ongoing sessions can be used to reinforce the teaching, and to assess the client's increasing skills and confidence in observing her fertility symptoms. There will be opportunities for discussing disturbances and other factors which affect the chart, including stress, illness, or medication.

Recording cervical changes

This optional indicator is not normally taught at the first session, to avoid confusion and overloading the client with information. Cervical palpation may be helpful for women experiencing difficulty observing the mucus symptom and particularly for women in special circumstances.

Use of the calendar calculation or later the Doering rule

These calculations can be introduced as additional indications of the onset of the fertile phase. Calculations are particularly useful for women who have difficulty in recognising the first appearance of cervical mucus.

Minor indicators of fertility

These confirmatory signs of fertility can be helpful. Women who suffer premenstrual symptoms may find that understanding their symptoms and their timing helps them to manage their lives. Women who suffer severe symptoms should be referred for treatment and advice.

Use of guidelines
Clients should be introduced to the guidelines appropriate to circumstances, considering the flexibility or strictness required, depending on their motivation. The importance of double check methods must be stressed.

Special circumstances
Post-natal mothers, women coming off the pill and pre-menopausal women will need additional support, and teaching appropriate to their circumstances. It is important that when women learn about their fertility during normal fertility, they understand the need for additional support at times of changing circumstances.

Flexibility of the teaching programme
During each session, time should be allowed for questions and for discussion. Clients with family planning, sexual or emotional problems, may find difficulty in expressing their feelings or anxieties and will need time and space to do so. The teaching format can be very flexible and should always be responsive to the needs of the client. Although this is an educational programme, the wider implications and practical use necessitate a counselling approach at all times. Most clients will be confident and autonomous in their use of NFP after about six months, but follow-up sessions should be offered at approximately nine months and then one year, thereafter offering additional support where cyclic change or changes in circumstances dictate.

CLIENT AUTONOMY
Before being considered independent in her use of NFP, the client should be able to:

Identify the length of cycle

Interpret the temperature chart:
- Day of shift.
- First day of the post-ovulatory infertile phase.

Interpret the mucus pattern:
- Onset of mucus.
- Different types of mucus.
- Identify peak day.
- Identify the fertile phase.

Apply a calculation:
- Shortest cycle minus 20.
- Doering rule.

Explain factors which may affect:
- The menstrual cycle.
- The temperature chart.
- The mucus pattern.

Apply the guidelines:
- To conceive.
- To avoid pregnancy.

In special circumstances, such as breast-feeding, post-pill or during the pre-menopausal years, the woman will need additional support and the teacher should be confident that the woman is able to interpret accurately the guidelines appropriate to her circumstances.

TEACHING RESOURCES

■ Fertility thermometers and digital thermometers.
■ Sympto-thermal charts.
■ Red, yellow and green highlight pens.
■ Client history sheets.
■ Client autonomy sheets.
■ User booklet with written instructions.
■ Flip-charts or overheads (prepared by the teacher) or
■ Appropriate video or slide programmes.

The teaching video *Fertility* is used by many NFP teachers to reinforce teaching and can also reduce teaching time. The programme is divided into six parts:
■ Anatomy and physiology – understanding human fertility.
■ The sympto-thermal method.
■ Achieving pregnancy.
■ For breast-feeding mothers.
■ After stopping the contraceptive pill.
■ NFP pre-menopause.
Couples can be shown the relevant part of the video at an appropriate time. The video can also be used in a group setting and as such can provide a useful means of promoting discussion. These resources can be obtained by NFP teachers from the Natural Family Planning Service.

MANAGEMENT OF THE CLIENT WITH A DIFFICULT CHART

When faced with a client with a difficult chart, it is useful to consider the following possibilities. The difficult chart could be due to poor teaching, poor observation or recording, or poor compliance. Additionally there may be a physiological reason for the unusual chart. Further support is always available for NFP teachers from more experienced tutors and medical advisers.

POOR TEACHING
Has the client received instruction appropriate to her educational level and her existing knowledge of fertility? Does she understand the rationale behind the instructions?

INACCURATE TEMPERATURE RECORDINGS
Technique must be reassessed.

POOR MUCUS SYMPTOM
Remember mucus symptom is a subjective assessment. There may be a delayed appearance at the vulva, resulting in a delay in identifying the onset of the fertile phase. Mucus symptoms may be misinterpreted. Check external factors including drugs, infection, lifestyle.

POOR CERVICAL SYMPTOMS

For most women this is the most difficult to learn. Although women should be informed of all changes, most women recognise only one or two, for example softening, opening or tilt. A minimum of three months is normally required for a woman to detect these changes accurately.

POOR COMPLIANCE

Are there external factors such as stress, illness, medication or travel affecting the chart? Are there other internal stressors such as commitment within the relationship, or other relationship difficulties? Do the couples have conflicting motives or ambivalence about a future pregnancy?

FERTILITY PROBLEMS

There may be a physiological cause for the problem chart either known or undiagnosed. A woman who is trying to conceive should be referred to her doctor if three consecutive cycles, with accurate observation and recording, have identified:

- A luteal phase of 10 days or less from the temperature shift to the onset of bleeding.
- A monophasic chart.
- Absence of Spinnbarkeit mucus.
- Inter-menstrual bleeding or spotting.

It is very important for the teacher to recognise her limits of expertise and the need for early referral.

SIGNS AND SYMPTOMS REQUIRING MEDICAL ADVICE

Disorders of bleeding

■ Mid-cycle bleeding or spotting	■ Irregular bleeding
■ Very heavy bleeding or flooding	■ Spotting after intercourse
■ Any bleeding after the menopause	■ Amenorrhoea apart from pregnancy

Breast changes – any reported change from normal:

■ Changes in shape and size	■ Persistent tenderness or pain
■ Discharge or bleeding from the nipple	■ Lumps in breast

Vaginal changes and sexual problems

■ Increased or abnormal discharge	■ Pain or bleeding after intercourse
■ Increased vaginal dryness	■ Painful intercourse
■ Vulval pain or irritation	■ Reduced libido

Any other physical, emotional or sexual problems causing anxiety

MANAGING THE CLIENT WITH AN UNPLANNED PREGNANCY

Teachers must face the fact that at some time one of their clients will become pregnant – A FAILURE. A teacher is responsible for her own standard of teaching, but she is not responsible for the behaviour of her clients. They may depart from the guidelines she has set them for a variety of reasons, such as the difficulty of abstinence, or because of stress in the relationship. Very rarely the method may have failed them. All unplanned pregnancies should be recorded and a careful assessment made as to whether this was a user failure, a method failure or a teacher related failure. An NFP teacher should seek the support of her supervisor at this time.

Whatever the cause of an unplanned pregnancy the teacher should continue to offer support. The couple can learn a great deal if they understand why the pregnancy occurred. Many couples who have had an unplanned pregnancy continue to use the method after the birth, finding it reliable and suited to their needs. An unplanned pregnancy does not necessarily mean an unwanted child. Without the support of an NFP teacher, self-taught users are usually devastated by an unplanned pregnancy. Uncertain of where they have gone wrong, they abandon the method, labelling it unreliable.

LIVING WITH NATURAL FAMILY PLANNING

Couples using natural family planning as a means of spacing or limiting their families are faced with times when they must abstain from intercourse in order to avoid pregnancy.

The word abstinence has very negative connotations. Some people prefer to use the term 'waiting'. Abstinence implies the denial of a pleasant experience. This is a misnomer, as the period of abstinence can be very positive and beneficial to the relationship. Abstinence forms a natural part of every marriage, at times of separation, illness or around the time of childbirth. Nevertheless, abstinence can be difficult, the common problems being sexual frustration and the denial of spontaneity.

Tensions created by abstinence can lead to marital disharmony. It is more likely to do so if the woman alone is responsible for charting and interpreting the charts and if she alone decides when intercourse should or should not take place. It is important that the man should be as knowledgeable about the method as the woman. He should be using natural family planning for valid reasons, such as his concern for his partner's health, from moral convictions, or from dislike of using other methods.

Every teacher of natural family planning should be aware of the problems of abstinence and should therefore make an opportunity for a couple to discuss their difficulties, experienced or anticipated. Those couples who are experiencing difficulties in adapting to periods of abstinence should be helped to find their own way of dealing with the problems. It may be a time for a couple to review their whole sexual relationship. The pattern of sexual behaviour may have to be altered to allow for periods of abstinence from intercourse. Couples should be able to express their feelings about their physical and emotional needs, especially at times when intercourse is not possible. Skin contact, caressing and body massage can be valuable means of expressing love. At times, many women, and, contrary to popular belief many men too, simply wish to be held and cuddled. It is sad that caressing is often almost synonymous with intercourse.

It is worth noting that psycho-sexual counsellors helping couples with various sexual difficulties, often use a technique first described by Masters and Johnson. This involves periods of abstinence for one or two weeks, with a carefully constructed programme concentrating on loving one another, communicating love by looking, holding, caressing, talking and kissing. When there are no expectations of performance, foreplay in the conventional sense can become a pleasurable end in itself. Following a period of abstinence, many couples report a heightened sense of pleasure in intercourse once more.

Enthusiasm develops among couples using natural family planning. Their communication improves as they learn about their fertility and they grow to understand how they can use this knowledge to plan their families. Every couple has a right to be taught about their fertility and to value this attribute. Using natural family planning, they will be independent and in control of their fertility.

Appendix

INFORMATION WHICH CAN BE GAINED FROM THE SYMPTO-THERMAL CHART

A fertility chart is a diagnostic aid, giving information concerning normal or abnormal function of the menstrual cycle, which is of use to doctors or nurses in general practice, family planning clinics and in fertility clinics.

For the normal fertile woman:
- A biphasic sympto-thermal chart confirms ovulation which occurs approximately 24–48 hours before the temperature rise.
- It identifies the fertile phase when sexual intercourse can lead to conception.
- It identifies the infertile phases when intercourse will not lead to conception. (This is the basis of the sympto-thermal method of natural family planning.)

For the woman experiencing fertility problems:
- A monophasic chart shows that there has been no ovulation in this cycle.
- The short cycle showing early ovulation, or the long cycle showing late ovulation, may highlight the mis-timing of intercourse. This commonly occurs with women who have been told that they should have intercourse on the 14th day or mid-cycle.
- The short luteal phase is significant. Fertilisation may occur but implantation does not occur if the luteal phase is less than eight days.
- The mucus symptom indicates the days of maximum fertility. These days occur immediately prior to ovulation and before the temperature shift.
- Changes in the cervix can confirm the days of maximum fertility. This is of particular value when mucus secretion is scanty, as may occur in women over the age of 35 years and others who have recently stopped hormonal contraception.
- Charting a cycle is of great assistance in the accurate timing of diagnostic tests.
- A 'Day 21 Progesterone' must be carried out some days after ovulation regardless of the day of cycle. Similarly a 'Sperm-Mucus Compatibility test' must be carried out when fertile mucus is present, prior to ovulation.

For the woman suffering from Pre-menstrual Syndrome (PMS):
- Diagnosis is confirmed by the timing and regularity of cyclical symptoms.
- Women with PMS often produce erratic temperature charts and abnormalities in the pattern of cervical mucus, which become normal as symptoms subside.

For the woman in the years of the pre-menopause:
- Declining fertility and symptoms of the pre-menopause can be monitored on the chart.
- Monophasic temperature charts (anovulatory cycles) give reassurance that delayed periods are not due to pregnancy.

Name

Shortest known cycle ☐ days
Length of this cycle ☐ days

Route of temperature
Time of taking temperature

O	V	R

	Month
	Date
	Day
°F	°C

Age

Chart Number

°F	°C
99.6	37.4
99.4	37.3
99.2	37.2
99.0	37.1
98.8	**37.0**
98.6	36.9
98.4	36.8
98.2	36.7
98.0	36.6
97.8	36.5
97.6	36.4
97.4	36.3
97.2	36.2
97.0	36.1
96.8	**36.0**
96.6	35.9
96.4	35.8
96.2	35.7
96.0	35.6
95.8	35.5

Special Notes/Disturbances

Sexual Intercourse (circle day of cycle)

1 2 3 4 5 6 7 8 9 10 11 12 13 14 15 16 17 18 19 20 21 22 23 24 25 26 27 28 29 30 31 32 33 34 35 36 37 38 39 40

Mucus-Sensation
Appearance
Stretch

Cyclical Symptoms

Cervix-Rising
Opening
Softening
Tilt

See instructions overleaf

Key

i	
P	Period or Blood Loss
D	Dry day
M	Mucus
F	Highly Fertile
⊠	Peak day

INSTRUCTIONS FOR USE OF THE SYMPTO-THERMAL CHART

Temperature

1. Shake the mercury down to below 35°C the night before.
2. Take the temperature immediately on waking, before getting out of bed or doing anything. If the recording time varies by more than one hour, note this on the chart.
3. Either (a) place the bulb of the thermometer under the tongue in contact with the floor of the mouth, close to the lips and leave for FIVE minutes, (b) insert the thermometer into the vagina for THREE minutes, (c) smear a trace of vaseline or KY jelly on the bulb and insert into the rectum for THREE minutes. (Any change in temperature-taking route should be made at the beginning of the cycle.)
4. Remove the thermometer, read it and mark on the chart with a dot in the centre of the appropriate square, not on the line. Join the dots to form a continuous graph.
5. If the mercury stops between two marks, take the lower reading.
6. Clean the thermometer with a little cotton wool and COLD water.
7. The first day of menstruation is day 1 of the cycle. Start a new chart on that day. If menstruation starts during the day, transfer that morning's temperature to a new chart.

Mucus

1. Mucus should be observed throughout the day and the chart marked each evening.
2. Mark each day of menstruation or blood loss including spotting with a P.
3. Mark each when there is no mucus with a D.
4. Mark days of sticky white/yellow mucus with an M.
5. Mark slippery/transparent/stretchy mucus with an F.
6. Mark peak day (LAST day of highly fertile 'egg-white' mucus) with a cross through F.
7. Use your own words to describe sensation, appearance and finger-test consistency of the mucus.

Cervix

1. Cervix during the infertile time: mark the cervix as a black circle placed low on the baseline, to show a low, firm, closed cervix ●. Draw a slanted line / below to show the tilt.
2. Cervix during the fertile time: use a clear circle to show the softening of the cervix ○ and an inner ring to show the cervix is open ◎. Place the symbol higher in the space provided to indicate the rising cervix. Draw a vertical line below to show the fertile cervix in position.

Sexual Intercourse Indicate intercourse by placing a circle round the appropriate day

Cyclical Symptoms Indicate cyclical symptoms, for example, mid-cycle pain, breast tenderness, abdominal bloating, rectal pressure and mood changes.

Disturbances Late nights, alcohol, illness, drugs, travel, other physical and emotional upsets, should be noted under the appropriate dates, and in Special Notes/Disturbances Box.

For further help or charts, contact:
The NFP Service, Clitherow House, 1 Blythe Mews, Blythe Road
London W14 0NW   Telephone 0171 371 1341

Your local NFP contact is:

Addresses

Natural Family Planning Service
Clitherow House
1 Blythe Mews
Blythe Road
London W14 ONW
Tel: 0171 371 1341
Fax: 0171 371 4921

National Association of Natural
Family Planning Teachers (NANF-
PT)
NFP Centre
Birmingham Maternity Hospital
Birmingham B15 2TG
Tel: 0121 627 2698

Billings Family Life Centre
58B Vauxhall Grove
London SW8 1TB
Tel: 0171 793 0026

Family Planning Association
27–35 Mortimer Street
London W1N 7RJ
Tel: 0171 636 7866

Graves Medical Audiovisual Library
Concord Video & Film Council Ltd
201 Felixstowe Road
Ipswich
Suffolk IP3 9BJ
Tel: 01473 726012

World Health Organisation
Geneva
Switzerland

Institute for Reproductive Health
Georgetown University School of
Medicine
2115 Wisconsin Avenue NW
Suite 602
Washington
DC 20007
USA

International Federation for Family
Life Promotion (IFFLP)
2009 N 14th Street
Suite 512
Arlington
VA 22201
USA

The Federation is in contact with
affiliated organisations in over 100
countries.

Australian Council of NFP
10th Floor
Polding House
276 Pitt Street
Sydney
NSW 2000
Australia

New Zealand Association of NFP
PO Box 36–329
Northcote
Auckland 9
New Zealand

SERENA Canada
6646 St Denis
Montreal
Quebec H26 2R9
Canada

Bibliography

NATURAL FAMILY PLANNING BOOKS

Billings, Dr Evelyn, and Westmore, Ann. *The Billings Method* (Penguin,1994)

Billings, Dr John J. *The Ovulation Method* (Advocate Press Ltd, Melbourne, Australia, 1983)

Flynn, Dr Anna, and Brooks, Melissa. *A Manual of Natural Family Planning* (George Allen & Unwin, 1990)

Menezes, Dr J. *Natural Family Planning in Pictures* (Catholic Hospital Association of India, 1982)

Roetzer, Dr Joseph. *Family Planning the Natural Way* (Fleming H. Revell Company, USA, 1981)

Shivanandan, Mary. *Natural Sex* (Hamlyn 1979)

Thyma, Paul. *The Double Check Method of Natural Family Planning* (Liturgical Press, 1978)

World Health Organisation. *Family Fertility Education, Teaching Package* (1982)

NFP ARTICLES

Consensus Statement. 'Breast-feeding as a Family Planning Method', *Lancet* Nov, 1988, pp1204-5

Howie, P. 'Natural regulation of fertility', *British Medical Bulletin* 1993, Vol 49. No 1, pp182-199

Report by Kathy Kennedy from an international group of scientists at the Bellagio Study & Conference Centre, Italy

NFP RESEARCH STUDIES

Barbato, M. and Bartolotti, M. 'Natural methods for fertility control, prospective study', *International Journal of Fertility and Sterility* 1988, No 5, Supplement, pp 48-51

Chretien, F. C., Cohen, J. et al. 'Human cervical mucus during the menstrual cycle and pregnancy in normal and pathological conditions', *Journal of Reproductive Medicine*, May 1975, Vol 14, No 5

Chretien, F.C. 'The cyclic variations of the spatial distribution of cervical mucus framework as demonstrated by scanning electron microscopy', *Scanning Electron Microscopy of Human Reproductive Physiology*, Acta Obstet Gynae Scand

Clubb, E.M., Pyper, C.M. and Knight, J. 'A pilot study on teaching natural family planning in general practice'

Collins, W.P., Branch, C. et al. 'Biochemical indices of the fertile period in women', *International Journal of Fertility*, 1981 26 (3), pp 196-202

Flynn, Docker, Morris, Lynch and Roberts. 'The reliability of women's subjective assessment of the fertile period, relative to urinary gonadotrophins and follicular ultrasonic measurements during the menstrual cycle', *Research in Family Planning* 1983

Frank-Herman, P, Freundl, G. et al. 'Effectiveness and acceptability of the sympto-thermal method of natural family planning in Germany', *Am J Obstet Gynecol* 1991, 165, pp2052-4

Graham, Gosling and France. 'An evaluation of teaching cervical mucus symptoms to ovulating infertile women', *Australian and New Zealand Journal of Obstetrics and Gynaecology* 1983

Gross, B. 'Breastfeeding and the return of fertility' (Endocrine Unit, Department of Medicine, Westmead Centre, NSW, Australia, 1983)

Keefe, E. F. 'Self-observation of the cervix to distinguish days of possible fertility', *Bulletin of the Sloane Hospital for Women* (Columbia, 1962)

Marshall, Prof John. 'Thermal changes in the normal menstrual cycle', *British Medical Journal* 1963, 1, p102

Marshall, Prof. John. 'A prospective trial of the mucothermic method of natural family planning', *International Review of Natural Family Planning*, Summer 1985

Marshall, Prof John, and Barrett, Dr John. 'The risk of conception on different days of the menstrual cycle', *Population Studies* 1969, Vol 23, p455

'Natural family planning: Current knowledge and new strategies for the 1990s' pp130-2 (Georgetown University, Washington DC 1990).

Odeblad, Prof Erik. 'The biophysical properties of the cervical-vaginal secretions', *International Review of Natural Family Planning* (St Johns, Collegeville, Minnesota, 1983)

Parenteau-Carreau, Dr Suzanne. 'The return of fertility in breast-feeding women', study of 54 breast-feeding experiences (1983)

Perez, A. 'First ovulation after childbirth', *American Journal of Obstetrics and Gynaecology* 1982

Perez, A., Labbok, M. and Queenan, J. 'Clinical study of the lactational amenorrhoea method for family planning', *Lancet* 1992, 339, pp968-70

RCGP oral contraceptive study 'Incidence of arterial disease among oral contraceptive users', *General Practitioner*, Vol 33, pp75-82

Rice, F.J., Lanctot, C. and Garcia-Devesa. 'Efficiency of the sympto-thermal method', *International Journal of Fertility* 1981, 26, pp222-30

Vessey, Martin, Smith and Yeates, Oxford, FPA study 'Return of fertility after discontinuance of oral contraceptives - influence of age and parity', *British Journal of Family Planning*, 1986, Vol 11, pp120-40

Wade, M. and McCarthy, P. 'Comparative study of ovulation and the sympto-thermal method', *American Journal of Obstetrics and Gynecology* 1981, 141, pp368-76

Weinberg and Wilcox. 'Using the ratio of urinary oestrogen and progesterone metabolites to estimate day of ovulation', *Statistics in medicine*, 10, pp255-66

'Models relating timing of intercourse to the probability of conception and the sex of the baby' (in press)

Wood, J.W. 'Fecundity and natural fertility in humans', *Oxford Review of Reproductive Biology* 1989, 11, 61-109

World Health Organisation studies. 'A prospective multi-center trial of the ovulation method of natural family planning', (The American Fertility Society, Birmingham, Alabama, USA, 1981-3)

   1 *The Teaching Phase* 1981, Vol 36 No 2

   2 *The Effectiveness Phase* 1981, Vol 36, No 5

   3 *Characteristics of the Menstrual Cycle and of the Fertile Phase* 1983, Vol 40, No 6

   4 *The Outcome of Pregnancy* 1984, Vol 41, No 4

BREAST-FEEDING

Renfrew, M., Fisher, C. and Arms, S. *Bestfeeding - Getting Breastfeeding Right for You* (Celestial Arts, 1990)

Rodriguez-Garcia, R. *Lactation Education for Health Professionals* (Pan American Health Organisation/Georgetown University, Washington DC, USA, 1990)

CONTRACEPTION

Freely, Maureen, and Pyper, Celia. *Pandora's Clock* (Cedar Press, 1994)

Guillebaud, Dr John. *The Pill* (Oxford University Press, 1994)

Loudon, Nancy. *Handbook of Family Planning* (Churchill Livingstone, 1985)

Mosse,J. and Heaton, J. *The Fertility and Contraception Book* (Faber and Faber, 1990)

SEXUALLY TRANSMITTED DISEASES

Adler, Michael. *ABC of Sexually Transmitted Diseases* (BMJ, 1992)

GYNAECOLOGY

McPherson, Ann (ed). *Women's Problems in General Practice* (Oxford University Press, 1990)

AUDIO-VISUAL PROGRAMMES

Natural Family Planning Parts 1-4, Sympto-thermal method, Breast-feeding and Pre-menopause tape-slide programmes (Concord Video and Film Council Ltd, Ipswich, Suffolk)

Clubb, Elizabeth and Knight, Jane. *A Guide to Natural Family Planning.* Video in six parts (produced and distributed by Oxford Medical Illustration, John Radcliffe Hospital, Oxford)

Glossary

Abortion Spontaneous or induced termination of pregnancy.

Abstinence Refraining from sexual intercourse. To avoid pregnancy, abstinence includes the avoidance of genital contact during the fertile phase of the cycle.

Adhesion Fibrous tissue that abnormally binds organs or other body parts, usually as a result of inflammation or abnormal healing of a surgical wound.

Amenorrhoea Absence of menstruation.
    Primary Complete absence of menstruation after puberty.
    Secondary Absence of menstruation for at least three months in a woman who has previously menstruated and is not pregnant or breast-feeding. Other causes include the contraceptive pill, stress, fatigue, psychological disturbance, obesity, weight loss, and anorexia nervosa.

Amniocentesis Puncture of the fluid sac surrounding the foetus to obtain a sample of the amniotic fluid for testing. Performed around the sixteenth week of pregnancy, the procedure can be used to diagnose neural tube defects, such as spina bifida, or genetic defects, such as Down's syndrome.

Androgens Male sex hormones, responsible for the development of male secondary sex characteristics including facial hair and a deep voice. Most androgens, including the principal one, testosterone, are produced in the testes. Small amounts are also produced in a woman's ovaries and adrenal glands.

Anovulation Absence of ovulation.

Anovulatory (anovular) cycle or episode 'Cycle' in which there is no ovulation, characterised by a monophasic chart.

Antibiotic Drug, for example penicillin, that is used to treat diseases caused by bacteria.

Antibody Specific protein substance produced by the body's immune (defence) system in response to an antigen (foreign substance), for example bacteria, which are rendered harmless.

Arousal fluid Colourless, lubricative fluid secreted around the vaginal opening in response to sexual stimulation, in preparation for intercourse.

Artificial insemination Insertion of seminal fluid into the vagina, cervix or uterus by means other than sexual intercourse. Sperm may be from the husband (AIH) or a donor (AID).

Assisted conception Any procedure where doctors assist with the conception process itself.

Bacteria Microscopic single-celled organisms. Some, known as commensals, live in or on the body without doing any harm and are beneficial to health, eg Doderlein's bacillae in the vagina. Pathogenic bacteria cause disease on entering the body, for example gonococcus causes gonorrhoea.

Bartholin's glands Small glands which produce the colourless lubricative arousal fluid around the vaginal opening in response to any sexual stimulation.

Basal body temperature (BBT) Temperature of the body at rest, taken immediately on waking, before any activity.

Basic infertile pattern (BIP) Positive sensation of dryness, with an absence of mucus or the presence of unchanging mucus (recognised as unchanging for at least two weeks initially). Indicates relative inactivity of the ovaries and low oestrogen levels, and may be recognised during very long cycles or during long periods of anovulation, such as during breast-feeding or pre-menopausally.

Billings method see Ovulation method.

Biopsy Removal of tissue from the body for microscopic examination and diagnosis.

Biphasic chart Two-phase temperature chart which shows a pattern of relatively low temperatures in the pre-ovulatory phase of the cycle, an upward shift of about 0.2°C confirming ovulation, and a sustained higher level until the next menstruation (ovulatory cycle).

Breast-feeding Process by which the baby is nourished from the mother's breasts. May take the form of full or nearly full breast-feeding, where the baby is nourished solely from the breasts; partial breast-feeding, where supplementary feeds or solids are given; and token breast-feeding, where the breast is used at irregular intervals, primarily for comfort rather than nourishment.

Calendar calculation Technique of calculating the pre-ovulatory relatively infertile phase based on previous cycle lengths (S minus 20 rule).

Calendar method Method of family planning in which the fertile phase of the cycle is calculated according to the length of at least six previous menstrual cycles.

Cervical crypts Complex pouches in the mucus-secreting lining of the cervix in which sperm may collect prior to ovulation.

Cervical ectropian (erosion) Condition of the cervix in which the mucus membrane lining the cervical canal turns outwards over the lip of the cervix. May result in a continuous mucus discharge. Also called cervical eversion.

Cervical mucus (secretion) Secretion from the cells lining the cervix, which changes under the influence of the female sex hormones.

Cervical mucus method see Ovulation method.

Cervical palpation Technique of self-examination of the cervix to determine the fertile and infertile phases of the cycle.

Cervical secretion see Cervical mucus.

Cervix Lower portion of the uterus that projects into the vagina.

Chromosome One of the 46 microscopic rod-shaped structures in a cell nucleus that carries the genetic information in the form of genes.

Chromosomes, sex Chromosomes in the human cell that determine the sex. Females have two 'X' chromosomes; males have one 'X' and one 'Y' chromosome.

Clitoris Small knob of very sensitive erectile tissue, situated where the labia unite at the front. Female counterpart of the male glans penis.

Coitus (intercourse) Complete sexual intercourse leading to ejaculation in the vagina – see Sexual intercourse.
    Coitus interruptus (withdrawal) Incomplete sexual intercourse in which the penis is deliberately withdrawn from the vagina so that ejaculation take places outside it.
    Coitus reservatus Sexual activity in which the penis is inserted into the vagina but ejaculation is deliberately avoided.

Colostrum First thick yellow milk secreted by the breasts in the last few weeks of pregnancy and the first two to three days after childbirth, until lactation is established. Colostrum contains high levels of protein, and antibodies.

Colposcopy Procedure used to examine the vagina and cervix under magnification through an instrument known as a colposcope. Of particular value in the early detection of cancer of the cervix.

Conceive To become pregnant.

Conception Fusion of the sperm and the egg cell.

Contraception Prevention of conception.

Corpus luteum (yellow body) Endocrine gland, formed in the ruptured follicle after ovulation, which produces progesterone. If the ovum (egg cell) is fertilised, the corpus luteum continues to produce hormones to support the early pregnancy. If fertilisation does not occur, the corpus luteum degenerates within 12–16 days.

Coverline Technique used for interpreting a temperature shift on the sympto-thermal chart.

Cowper's glands Pair of small glands in the male which secrete the lubricative pre-ejaculatory fluid.

Crypts see Cervical crypts.

CVS (chorionic villus sampling) Antenatal test involving a needle aspiration through the uterus to obtain a sample of the placental tissue. Used to detect genetic or spinal defects, if there are high risk factors present.

Cyst Abnormal sac-like structure containing fluid or semi-solid material, which may present as a lump in various parts of the body. Most cysts are benign (non-malignant) but some may become cancerous (malignant). All lumps require medical assessment.

Dilatation and curettage (D and C) Surgical procedure used to scrape the surface of the endometrium with an instrument called a curette. Prior to curettage, the cervix is gradually opened with instruments called dilators.

Doering rule Calculation to determine the first fertile day of the cycle based on the earliest previous temperature shift.

Double-check method Method of natural family planning using the temperature, cervical mucus, cervical palpation and calendar calculation to ensure a check of at least two indicators. The double check need not include temperature readings, for example a woman may rely on mucus and cervical symptoms as a double check.

Douche Cleansing fluid flushed through the vagina as a hygienic measure. Unnecessary practice which should be strongly discouraged.

Dysmenorrhoea Painful menstruation due to spasmodic contractions of the uterus, usually arising just prior to or for the first few hours of menstruation, then gradually subsiding.

Dyspareunia Painful or difficult intercourse.

Ectopic pregnancy Implantation and development of a fertilised ovum outside the uterus, usually in the fallopian tube.

Effectiveness Measure of the efficiency of a family planning method in avoiding pregnancy.
  Method effectiveness Measure of the effectiveness of a family planning method under ideal conditions, when used according to the instructions. Also referred to as the theoretical or biological effectiveness.
  Use effectiveness Measure of the effectiveness of a method of family planning under real-life conditions. Often referred to as the practical or behavioural effectiveness.

Ejaculation Release of seminal fluid from the penis during male orgasm.

Embryo Initial stages of development of the unborn child, from the fertilised egg to around eight weeks after conception.

Endometriosis Growth of endometrial tissue in areas other than the uterus, for example the fallopian tubes or the ovaries. May contribute to fertility problems.

Endometrium Inner lining of the uterus which is shed during menstruation. If conception occurs, the fertilised egg implants in the endometrium.

Fallopian tube One of a pair of tubes through which the ripened ovum is transported from the ovary towards the uterus. In the fertile phase, sperm may pass from the uterus towards the outer end of the fallopian tube, where fertilisation normally takes place.

Family planning Methods used by sexually active couples to prevent, space or achieve pregnancy in order to attain the desired family size.

Ferning (Fern test) Characteristic ferning pattern shown by highly oestrogenised fertile mucus when dried on a glass slide.

Fertile phase Days of the menstrual cycle during which sexual intercourse may result in pregnancy – see Fertility cycle.

Fertilisation Fusion of a sperm with an ovum, normally in the outer end of the fallopian tube.

Fertility Ability of a couple to reproduce.

Fertility awareness Essential basic education for understanding fertility throughout reproductive life.

Fertility cycle Can be divided into two phases: the phase before ovulation, the pre-ovulatory or follicular phase; and the phase after ovulation, the post-ovulatory or luteal phase. For natural family planning purposes, the cycle is often divided into three significant phases.
    The pre-ovulatory relatively infertile phase (early infertile phase) starts at the onset of menstruation and ends at the onset of the fertile phase.
    The fertile phase includes the time of ovulation and the days before and after ovulation, when intercourse may result in pregnancy.
    The post-ovulatory infertile phase (late infertile phase) starts at the completion of the fertile phase and ends at the onset of the next menstruation.

Fibroid Benign fibrous and muscular growth of tissue in the muscular wall of the uterus.

Foetus Unborn child from around eight weeks after conception (when all major organs are formed and it begins to resemble a human being) to the time of birth.

Follicle Small fluid-filled structure in the ovary which contains the ovum or egg cell.

Follicle-stimulating hormone (FSH) Pituitary hormone that stimulates the ripening of follicles in the ovary, and the production of the ovarian hormone oestrogen. In the male, FSH regulates the formation of sperm in the testes.

Follicular phase Pre-ovulatory phase characterised by the growth and development of the egg follicles – see Menstrual cycle and Pre-ovulatory phase.

Gamete Mature male or female sex cell – the sperm or ovum.

Genes Basic unit of genetic material which is carried at a particular place on a chromosome.

Genetic Relating to hereditary characteristics.

Genital contact Contact between the penis and the vulva without penetration.

Genitals (genitalia) Reproductive organs of either the male or female. Usually refers to the external parts of the reproductive system – see Vulva.

Gonads Primary sex glands – testes (male) and ovaries (female).

Hormone Chemical substance which is produced and secreted by an endocrine (ductless) gland. The hormone is carried by the blood to a target organ where it exerts its effect. For example, follicle-stimulating hormone is produced in the pituitary gland and travels via the blood to the ovary, where it stimulates the growth and maturation of follicles.

Hot flush Sudden flash of heat particularly affecting the face, neck and chest and lasting from a few seconds to several minutes. May spread over the upper part of the body and be accompanied by sweating. Most commonly due to low oestrogen levels related to the pre-menopause.

Human chorionic gonadotrophin (HCG) One of the main hormones unique to pregnancy, produced by the developing embryo from its earliest days. Main action is to maintain the corpus luteum and hence the secretion of oestrogen and progesterone until the placenta has developed sufficiently to take over hormonal production – see Pregnancy test.

Hysterectomy Surgical removal of the uterus.

Implantation Process by which the fertilised egg embeds in the endometrium.

Infertile phase Days of the menstrual cycle during which intercourse cannot result in pregnancy – see Fertility cycle.

Infertility Inability of a couple to reproduce.

Intercourse see Coitus, Sexual intercourse.

Inter-menstrual bleeding Appearance of bleeding, spotting or a brownish mucus discharge between two menstrual periods. Indicates the need for medical assessment.

In-vitro fertilisation (IVF) Method of assisted conception in which fertilisation takes place in a glass dish (vitro=glass). Sometimes referred to as the 'test-tube baby' technique.

Labia Folds of skin which form the inner lips (labia minora) and outer lips (labia majora) on both sides of the vaginal opening, making up part of the female external genitals.

Lactation Production and secretion of milk by the breasts – see Breast-feeding.

Lactational amenorrhoea method (LAM) Natural method of family planning for breast-feeding mothers, which recognises that breast-feeding suppresses fertility during the first six months post-partum, provided that the mother is fully breast-feeding and is amenorrhoeic.

Laparoscopy Surgical procedure used to view the abdominal organs through an illuminated instrument known as a laparoscope. May be used for examination of the ovaries and fallopian tubes in infertility investigations, and for other gynaecological operations including female sterilisation.

Libido Sexual drive. Frequently refers to the intensity of sexual desires.

Lochia Blood-stained discharges from the uterus for the first few weeks after childbirth.

Luteal phase Post-ovulatory phase characterised by the growth and development of the corpus luteum – see Menstrual cycle, Post-ovulatory phase.

Luteinising hormone (LH) Hormone from the pituitary gland that stimulates ovulation and the development of the corpus luteum.

Menarche First menstrual period a girl experiences at the start of reproductive life.

Menopause Last menstrual period a woman experiences at the end of reproductive life.

Menstrual cycle Cycle of physiological changes in the ovaries, cervix and endometrium under the influence of the female sex hormones. The length of the menstrual cycle is calculated from the first day of menstrual bleeding to the day before the following menstruation. The term fertility cycle may be used in place of menstrual cycle, emphasising the fertility aspect – see Fertility cycle.

Menstruation, menses, menstrual period Cyclic shedding of the endometrium, consisting of blood, mucus and cellular debris. Normally occurs about two weeks after ovulation.

Minor indicators of fertility Physical and emotional changes, including Mittelschmerz pain, breast tenderness and mood changes, which may provide further signs of fertility.

Miscarriage or spontaneous abortion Premature and spontaneous expulsion of the embryo or foetus from the uterus.

Mittelschmerz (ovulation) pain One-sided sharp pain or dull ache in the lower abdomen occurring around the time of ovulation.

Mixed method use Combined use of barrier methods and fertility awareness. To avoid pregnancy, barrier methods are used during the fertile phase.

Monophasic chart Temperature chart which does not show the typical biphasic pattern. Temperature readings will be on one level, indicating an absence of ovulation.

Mucothermic method Natural method combining cervical mucus and temperature recordings.

Mucus see Cervical mucus.

Multiple index methods Natural family planning methods in which several indicators of fertility are used to detect the fertile and infertile phases of the cycle.

Natural family planning (NFP) Methods for planning or preventing pregnancy by observation of the naturally occurring signs and symptoms of the fertile and infertile phases of the menstrual cycle. To avoid pregnancy, couples using natural family planning methods abstain from intercourse during the fertile phase of the woman's menstrual cycle. (WHO definition). Lactational amenorrhoea method (LAM) is included as a natural method, even though it does not require abstinence from intercourse. Natural methods do not include coitus interruptus or the use of drugs, devices or surgical procedures to avoid pregnancy. Couples who combine barrier methods with fertility awareness are generally referred to as mixed method users – see Lactational amenorrhoea method, Mixed method use.

Oestrogen Hormone produced mainly by the ovaries which is responsible for female sexual development and female secondary sex characteristics. Increasing oestrogen levels in the follicular phase (pre-ovulatory phase) of the cycle stimulate significant changes in the cervix, cervical mucus, and endometrium.

Orgasm Climax of sexual excitement in the male or female. Ejaculation usually accompanies male orgasm. Occurrence of female orgasm is more variable, dependent upon both physiological and psychological factors.

Ovary One of a pair of female sex glands which produce ova and the female sex hormones oestrogen and progesterone. These hormones control the menstrual cycle and female secondary sex characteristics.

Ovulation Release of a mature ovum or egg cell from the ovarian follicle.

Ovulation method Technique of natural fertility control developed by Drs John and Evelyn Billings, in which days of infertility, possible fertility, and maximal fertility are identified by a woman's observations of mucus at the vulva. Sometimes referred to as the cervical mucus or cervical secretion method. The Creighton model is a variation, using a scoring system to grade types of mucus.

Ovulatory cycle Cycle in which ovulation occurs, characterised by a biphasic temperature chart.

Ovum Mature female sex cell, or egg (plural: ova).

Peak mucus day Last day when highly fertile mucus characteristics are either seen or felt. Can only be recognised in retrospect. Coincides closely with ovulation.

Pearl index Statistical measurement of contraceptive effectiveness, showing the number of pregnancies per 100 women-years of use, ie how many women would get pregnant if 100 women used a given method of family planning for one year.

Pelvic inflammatory disease Infection involving inflammation of female reproductive organs, particularly the fallopian tubes and ovaries. Pelvic infection resulting in tubal damage may be a cause of infertility.

Penis External male reproductive organ through which seminal fluid and urine can pass.

Perineum Area of tissue between the vulva and anus. The procedure of cutting this to enlarge the vaginal opening is known as episiotomy.

Period see Menstruation.

Periodic abstinence Method(s) of family planning based on voluntary avoidance of intercourse by a couple during the fertile phase of the cycle in order to avoid pregnancy.

Pituitary gland 'Master' endocrine (ductless) gland at the base of the brain that produces many important hormones, some of which trigger other glands into making their own hormones. Functions include hormonal control of the sex glands (ovaries and testes).

Planned or intended pregnancy Pregnancy which is consciously planned.

Post-ovulatory (luteal) phase Phase from ovulation to the onset of the next menstruation. Length is relatively constant, usually lasting 12–16 days.

Pre-ejaculatory fluid Small amount of lubricating fluid which is discharged involuntarily from the penis during sexual excitement, prior to ejaculation. May contain viable sperm.

Pregnancy Condition of nurturing the embryo or foetus within the woman's body, lasting from conception to birth. Normal duration is 265 days from conception to birth, or the more usual calculation of 280 days (40 weeks) from the first day of the last menstrual period.

Pregnancy test Early-morning urine sample is tested for the presence of human chorionic gonadotrophin (HCG), the pregnancy hormone. A positive result, indicating pregnancy, may be seen within several days of the missed period – see Human chorionic gonadotrophin.

Pre-menopause Period of months or years preceding the menopause, during which time there may be physical and emotional changes, including irregularities in the menstrual cycle, as a result of decreasing oestrogen and progesterone levels.

Pre-menstrual syndrome Collection of physical and emotional signs and symptoms which appear during the post-ovulatory phase and disappear at the onset of menstruation.

Pre-ovulatory (follicular) phase Variable-length phase from the onset of menstruation to ovulation.

Progesterone Hormone produced mainly by the corpus luteum in the ovary following ovulation, which prepares the endometrium for a possible pregnancy. Also responsible for the rise in basal body temperature, for changing the cervix to its infertile state and for changing the cervical mucus to form an impenetrable barrier to sperm.

Prolactin Pituitary hormone which stimulates the production of breast milk and inhibits the ovarian production of oestrogen.

Prostate gland Gland situated at the base of the male bladder. Its nutritive secretions add volume to make up the seminal fluid.

Puberty Time of life in boys and girls when the reproductive organs become functional and the secondary sexual characteristics appear.

Rhythm method – see Calendar method.

Scrotum Pouch of skin containing the testes which helps to regulate their temperature.

Secondary sex characteristics Features of masculinity or femininity that develop at puberty, under hormonal control.
  Male Deep voice and growth of beard, underarm and pubic hair, influenced by androgens.
  Female Rounding of the breasts, waist and hips, and growth of underarm and pubic hair, influenced by oestrogens.

Seminal fluid (semen) Viscous fluid ejaculated from the penis at orgasm. Contains sperm and secretions from the seminal vesicles and prostate gland.

Seminal vesicles Two sacs which open into the top of the male urethra. Secretions from these vesicles form part of the seminal fluid.

Sexual intercourse (coitus) Sexual activity during which the erect penis is inserted into the vagina where ejaculation takes place – see Coitus.

Sexually transmitted diseases Any infection that is transmitted by sexual contact or intercourse.

Single index method Natural family planning method in which only one indicator of fertility is used to detect the fertile and infertile phases of the cycle.

Sperm, spermatozoon Mature male sex cell (plural: spermatozoa). Sperm survive for 3–5 days in fertile cervical mucus.

Spinnbarkeit Elasticity or stretchiness characteristic of highly fertile mucus.

Spotting Small amounts of red or brownish discharge occurring during the menstrual cycle at times other than the true menstrual period – see Inter-menstrual bleeding.

Stop bar Short vertical line used on the chart to define the onset of the fertile phase by calculation.

Subfertility State of reduced fertility.

Sympto-thermal method (symptoms plus temperature) Natural method of family planning combining cervical mucus symptoms, a calendar calculation, optional cervical palpation and minor indicators of fertility, with temperature readings. Where temperature readings are not available, a double check method can be used.

Temperature chart Graph showing variation in daily basal body temperature – see Biphasic chart, Monophasic chart.

Temperature method Method of natural family planning in which the post-ovulatory infertile phase of the menstrual cycle is identified by a sustained rise in basal body temperature.

Temperature shift Rise in basal body temperature (of around 0.2°C) which divides the early low phase temperatures from the later higher phase temperatures on a biphasic chart.

Testicle (testis) One of a pair of male sex glands which produce sperm and the male sex hormones or androgens, including testosterone (plural: testes).

Testosterone Hormone produced by the testes, responsible for the development of male secondary sex characteristics and functioning of the male reproductive organs.

Ultrasound Diagnostic technique which uses sound waves to produce an image of internal body structures.

Unplanned or unintended pregnancy Pregnancy that the couple did not intend and which occurred despite the use of a family planning method to avoid pregnancy.

Urethra Tube which conveys urine from the bladder to the outside. The female urethra is very short, extending from the bladder to the urinary opening at the vulva. The male urethra is longer, extending along the length of the penis. It also conveys the seminal fluid.

Uterus (womb) Pear-shaped muscular organ in which the fertilised ovum implants and grows for the duration of pregnancy. Muscular contractions of the uterus push the infant out through the birth canal at the time of birth. If implantation does not occur, the uterine lining (endometrium) is shed at menstruation.

Vagina Muscular canal extending from the cervix to the opening at the vulva. Sperm are deposited in the vagina during intercourse. It is also through this canal that the baby is delivered (birth canal).

Vaginal discharge Any secretion which comes from the vagina, apart from menstrual bleeding (which originates in the uterus). Discharge may be normal (physiological) or abnormal (pathological).

Physiological discharges include mucus from the cervix, and clear fluid secreted by the vaginal walls and Bartholin's glands during sexual excitement.

Pathological discharges are distinguished by their unusual colour and unpleasant odour. May cause itching, irritation, soreness or burning of the vagina and vulva.

Vas deferens One of a pair of tubes which convey the seminal fluid from the testis to the urethra.

Vulva External female genitals comprising the two sets of labia (outer and inner lips) and the clitoris.

Zygote (fertilised ovum) Single fertilised cell resulting from fusion of the sperm and the egg cell. After further cell division the zygote is known as the embryo.

Index

Abdominal
  bloating, 63
  pain, 62
Abortion
  induced (termination of
  pregnancy), 120, 142–4,
  176
  spontaneous
  (miscarriage), 121–2, 176
Abstinence, 76,166–7, 176
Adhesions, 120, 176
Adolescence, 25, 39
Adrenal, glands,104–5
AIDS, 148–50
Alcohol, 34, 52, 53, 57, 118
Amenorrhoea, 121, 133, 176
Amniocentesis, 176
Anaemia, 110
Androgens, 176
Anorexia nervosa, 55, 121
Anovulatory (Anovular)
  cycles, 39, 176
  infertility, 123, 124, 126
  post-partum, 87
  post-pill, 96
  pre-menopause, 104, 110,
  114–6
Antibiotics, 56, 176
Arousal fluid, 28, 176
Artificial insemination, AIH
  and AID, 124–5, 177
Autonomous users, 163
Avoiding pregnancy, see
  guidelines

Barrier methods, 136–40
Bartholin's glands, 28, 177
Basal body temperature
  (BBT), 33–4, 177
Basic infertile pattern, 87,
  111, 177
Billings method, 10, 44, 74,
  177
Bioself thermometer, 158
Biphasic chart, 34–5, 168,
  177
Birth defects, 158
Bladder, 15, 16, 20
Bleeding
  inter-menstrual, 62
  post-natal, 87

post-pill, 97
pre-menopausal, 106,
  111, 114
vaginal, 24, 50
withdrawal, 97
Bottle feeding, effects on
  fertility, 94
Breast
  awareness, 108
  cancer, 108, 131
  tenderness, discomfort,
  62, 64–5
Breast-feeding, 82–4, 177
  fertility, and, 84–93

Calendar
  calculation, 66–7, 177
  method, 10, 13, 66, 178
Cancer
  breast, 108, 131
  cervical, 108, 131, 151
  endometrial, 108, 130,
  151
  ovarian, 130
Candidiasis (thrush), 145–6
Cap, cervical, 137
Cervical
  crypts, 18, 21, 26, 41, 178
  ectropian (erosion), 56,
  178
  mucus, 26–7, 41–51, 178
  secretions, see mucus
  smear, 108, 131, 151
Cervix, 178
  cyclical changes, 58–60
  incompetent, 122, 144
  self-examination of,
  59–60
Change of life, 103
Childbirth, fertility after,
  82–94
Chlamydia infections, 120,
  146
Chromosomes, 178
  sex, male and female,
  23–4, 156, 178
Clitoris, 19, 178
Clomiphene (Clomid), 126
Coitus, 178
  interruptus, 18, 178,
  184

reservatus, 178
Colour code, 69, 89, 112,
  162
Conception, 70–1, 179
  chances of, 70, 152–3
Condom
  female, 138–9
  male, 138
Cone biopsy, 121, 151
Contraception and
  sterilisation, 128–142, 179
Contraceptive pill
  combined, 95–7, 129–131
  coming off the, 95–102
  progestogen only, 131–2
Contraceptive system,
  personal, 157
Corpus luteum, 21–3, 179
Cost-effectiveness of NFP, 80
Coverline, 35, 179
  technique, 36, 90, 98–101,
  113, 115
Cowpers glands, 16, 17, 179
Creighton model, 45
Crypts, see cervical
CVS, chorionic villus
  sampling, 179
Cyst, 179
Cystitis, 106, 150

Depression, 64, 107
Diagnostic value of chart,
  168–9
Diaphragm, 136–7
Diet
  menopausal women, 108
  pre-conceptual, 118–19
  pre-menstrual syndrome,
  65
Disturbances, 52–3
Doering rule, 67, 179
Double check method, 11,
  32, 179
Drugs
  effects on the cycle, 55–6
  fertility, 126
Dysmenorrhoea, 64, 180
Dyspareunia, 106, 150, 180

Ectopic pregnancy, 120,
  132, 136, 180

Effectiveness, 180
  method, 77–8, 180
  use, 77–8, 180
  of contraception, 77
  of natural family
  planning, 77–81
Ejaculation, 16, 17, 180
Emergency contraception,
  140–1
Emotional changes, 62–5
Endometriosis, 121, 180
Endometrium, 21, 24–5,
  180
Erection, 18

Fallopian tubes, 21–3, 180
  infertility, 118, 120, 126
  sterilisation, 142
Fern test, 125, 154, 180
Fertile phase, 29–31, 43, 73,
  180
Fertilisation, 23, 181
Fertility, 181
  awareness, 12–14, 181
  cycle, 30–31, 181
Fever, 55
Fibroids,121, 181
Fimbriae, 22–3
Foetus, 119, 181
Follicles, 21, 181
  rupture of, *see* ovulation
  unruptured, *see* LUF
  syndrome
Follicle stimulating
  hormone, FSH, 28–9, 181
Follicular phase, 28–9, 181

Gamete, 181
Genes, 23, 181
Genital contact, 17, 182
Genitals, 182
  female, 18–20, 182
  male, 15–16, 182
Glans penis, 16, 19
Glass of water test, 50, 111
Gonads, 182
Gonorrhoea, 147
Group teaching, 159
Guidelines, normal fertility
  to avoid pregnancy, 72–3
  to conceive, 70–1
  breast-feeding, 90
  post-pill, 98–9
  pre-menopause, 115

Hepatitis B, 150
Herpes, genital, 147
History of NFP, 10–11

HIV, *see* AIDS
Hormone replacement
  therapy, HRT, 108–9
Hormones, sex, 28–30, 125,
  182
Hot flushes,106, 182
Human Chorionic
  Gonadotrophin, HCG, 25,
  182
Human Fertilisation and
  Embryology Act, HFEA,
  143
Hymen, 19–20
Hysterectomy, 182

Idiopathic infertility, 121
Illness, effects on the
  menstrual cycle, 55–7
Implantation, 23–4, 182
Implant, contraceptive, 133
Infertile phase, *see* fertility
  cycle
Infertility, 118–27, 182
Injectable contraceptives,
  132
Intercourse, sexual, 18, 182
Inter-menstrual bleeding,
  62, 111,182
Inter-menstrual pain, 62
Intra-uterine device, IUD,
  135
Intra-uterine system, IUS,
  134
In-vitro fertilisation, IVF,
  126, 182

Kegel exercise, 51

Labia, 18–19, 183
Lactational Amenorrhoea
  Method, LAM, 84–6, 183
Lactation, *see also* breast-
  feeding, 183
Laparoscopy, 125, 183
Libido, 63, 183
Life or death rules
  (Roetzer), 73
Living with NFP, 166–7
Lochia, 87, 183
Luteal phase, 30, 39, 168,
  183
Luteinised unruptured
  follicle syndrome, LUF,
  121
Luteinising hormone LH,
  28–30, 183
  test kits, 123
Lymph node sign, 63

Male reproductive organs,
  15–18
Medication – effects on
  cycle, 55, 56
Menarche, 25, 183
Menopause, 25, 104, 183
Men's role,12–14, 76, 160,
  166
Menstrual cycle, 24, 29,
  30–1, 183
Menstruation, 24, 183
Minor indicators of fertility,
  62–5, 184
Miscarriage, 121–2, 184
Mittlelschmerz pain, 62,
  184
Mixed method use, 140, 184
Modified mucus method,
  74–5
Monophasic chart, 39, 110,
  168, 184
Motivation, 76, 165
Muco-thermic method 11,
  184
Mucus, cervical, 26, 41–50,
  153–4, 184
  observation of, 41–44
  recording, 46–9
Multiple index methods, 11,
  184

Natural family planning,
  184
Non-specific urethritis,
  NSU, 146

Oestrogen, 21, 28–9, 84,
  104–5, 184
Orgasm, 184
  female, 19
  male, 18
Os, cervical (opening), 26,
  58–9, 87
Osteoporosis, 107
Ovarian monitor,157
Ovary, 21, 185
Ovulation, 21–2, 29, 185
  detection kits, 123, 157–8
  method, 10, 44–5, 74–5,
  78, 185
  pain, *see* Mittelschmerz
Ovulatory cycles, 34, 90, 96,
  110, 185
Ovum (pl. ova), 21–4, 185

Peak day, 43, 44, 46, 48–9,
  185
Peak, double, 53, 54,

Pearl index, 77, 185
Pelvic inflammatory
 disease, 146, 150, 120,
 185
Penetration, 18
Penis, 18
Peri-menopause, 104–5
Perineum, 19–20
Periodic abstinence, 185
Period, *see* menstruation
 pains, *see* dysmenorrhoea
Personal contraceptive
 system, 157
Pill, *see* contraceptive
Pituitary, gland, 28–9, 84,
 185
Post-coital contraception,
 see emergency
Post-ovulatory phase, 30,
 73, 80, 90, 99, 115, 186
Pre-conceptual care,
 118–19
Pre-ejaculatory fluid, 17–18,
 186
Pregnancy, 186
 achievement of, 70–1,
 118, 122
 avoidance of, 72–3
 planned (intended), 70,
 102, 118, 186
 test, 71, 186
 unplanned (unintended),
 166, 186
Pre-menopause, 104, 106–7
 169, 186
Pre-menstrual syndrome,
 PMS, 63–5, 169, 186
Pre-ovulatory phase, 28, 43,
 72,79, 90, 99, 115, 186
Progesterone, 21, 29–30, 33,
 186
 assays, 125, 168
Progestogen-only pill, 97,
 131–2
Progesturine TM PDG, 157
Prolactin, 84, 125, 186
Proliferative phase, 25–9
Prostate, gland, 16, 186
Puberty, 15, 25, 187

Reproductive system
 female, 18–31
 male, 15–18
Research, 77–81, 152–8
Rhythm method, *see*
 calendar method
Risk-taking, 141
.Rite Time thermometer, 157

Rubella, 118
Rugae, vaginal, 27
Rule of 3 over 6, 35
Rules, *see* guidelines

Saliva tests, 158
Scrotum, 15–16, 187
Secondary sex
 characteristics
 female, 21, 187
 male, 21,187
Secretory phase, 25, 29
Seminal fluid, semen,
 15–16, 187
Seminal vesicles, 16, 187
Sex determination, 24, 156–7
Sexual intercourse, 187
Sexually transmitted
 diseases, 145–50, 187
Sheath, *see* condom
Shift, 46, 62, 111; 187
Shortest cycle minus 20
 rule, 66–7, 69, 72
Single index methods, 10,
 187
S minus 20 rule, 66–7
Sperm, 17, 187
 antibodies, 125, 142
 count, normal values, 124
 penetration in mucus,
 125
 production, 15–16
 survival, 18
Spermicides, 139–40
Spinnbarkeit, 42, 43, 154,
 187
Spotting, 46, 62, 111; 187
Sterilisation
 female, 120–1, 142
 male, 124–5, 141–2
Stop-bar, 67, 69, 187
Stress, 53–5, 89, 103, 121
Subfertility, 118, 187
Sympto-thermal
 chart, 170, 171
 method, 32, 187
Syphilis, 148

Teaching fertility awareness
 and NFP, 11, 159–67
Teaching NFP in general
 practice, 80
Teaching resources, 164
Technological devices, 11,
 142, 157–8
Temperature
 basal body, 33
 factors affecting, 37, 52–7

interpreting readings,
 34–40
 method, 10, 188
 recording and charting,
 34, 188
 shift, 34–7, 188
Termination of pregnancy,
 142–4
Testicles, testes, 15–16, 120,
 188
Testosterone, 15, 188
Thermometer
 computerised, 157–8
 digital, 33, 161
 fertility (mercury), 33,
 161
Thrombosis, pill and, 131
Thrush, *see* candidiasis
Travel, effect on cycle, 52,
 57
Trichomoniasis, 146
True period, 97, 111
Tubal damage, 120, 142
Tubal ligation, *see*
 sterilisation, female,
Twins, 23

Ultrasound, 155–6, 188
Urethra,
 female, 19–20, 188
 male, 15–16, 188
Uterus, 20–21, 24–5, 188

Vagina, 27–8, 188
 acidity of, 27, 50
 discharge, 28, 145, 150,
 188
 dryness, 28, 106
 hygiene, 50
 infections, 145–6
 irritants, feminine
 lubrication, 28
Vaginitis, 106
Vas deferens, 16, 141–2, 189
Vasectomy, 141–2
Vitamins
 pre-menopause, 108
 pre-menstrual, 65
Vulva, 18–20, 189

Warts, genital, 147
Weaning, 89, 91, 93
Well Woman clinics, 107–8
WHO studies, 78
Withdrawal, *see* coitus
 interruptus

Zygote, 23, 189